Praise for *Storied Companions*

"In the right hands, Buddhist narratives can offer us abundant and consequential lessons about how to live and how to die. After reading this nuanced, layered, tender, and courageous book, we are left feeling profound gratitude. Because of Karen Derris's deep practice of reading and retelling Buddhist stories, we can clearly sense that she is 'looking over her shoulder,' extending to us her hand, and encouraging us to orientate our lives by love rather than by fear. This is an amazing gift, one beyond measure."—Jan Willis, author of *Dreaming Me: Black, Baptist, and Buddhist* and *Dharma Matters: Women, Race, and Tantra*

"Karen Derris writes of her journey through life, cancer, and facing death with such eloquence in *Storied Companions*. Often paired with Buddhist narratives, she tells how living with an open heart is possible even when living with a terminal illness. This is a touching and inspirational book."—Sharon Salzberg, author of *Lovingkindness* and *Real Change*

"This book holds an astonishing combination of hard reality with visionary light and love. Neither cancels out the other. The result is a gift to its readers, teaching us how to see our own reality, whatever that might be; teaching us how to place ourselves directly into stories of great profundity from Buddhist tradition; and teaching us how to read our own life stories through the lucid lens of honesty with which Derris tells us hers. This is a book of great compassion and clarity."—Janet Gyatso, Hershey Professor of Buddhist Studies, Harvard Divinity School

"There are many miracles in Karen Derris's life. Not the least of which is this shimmering memoir. Reading the life story of this smart, compassionate scholar and writer, as intellectually bold as she is physically courageous, I learned how the great Buddhist stories reflect and intermingle with the most profound human experiences. This is a book about love in its infinite manifestations. In the face of daunting circumstances, Derris's voice is sweet and strong, an aria of benevolence. Reading *Storied Companions* made me want to be a better person."
—Leslie Brody, author of *Sometimes You Have to Lie: The Life and Times of Louise Fitzhugh, Renegade Author of* Harriet the Spy

Storied Companions

Cancer, Trauma, and Discovering Guides
for Living in Buddhist Narratives

Karen Derris

FOREWORD BY HIS HOLINESS THE SEVENTEENTH KARMAPA

Wisdom Publications
199 Elm Street
Somerville, MA 02144 USA
wisdomexperience.org

Library of Congress Cataloging-in-Publication Data
Names: Derris, Karen, author.
Title: Storied companions: cancer, trauma, and discovering guides for living in
   Buddhist narratives / Karen Derris; foreword by his holiness the Seventeenth
   Karmapa.
Description: First. | Somerville: Wisdom Publications, 2021. |
   Includes bibliographical references.
Identifiers: LCCN 2020051300 (print) | LCCN 2020051301 (ebook) |
   ISBN 9781614295754 (paperback) | ISBN 9781614295990 (ebook)
Subjects: LCSH: Suffering—Religious aspects—Buddhism. | Life—Religious
   aspects—Buddhism. | Death—Religious aspects—Buddhism. | Buddhist stories.
   | Tibetan Buddhism.
Classification: LCC BQ4235 .D47 2021 (print) | LCC BQ4235 (ebook) |
   DDC 204/.42—dc23
LC record available at https://lccn.loc.gov/2020051300
LC ebook record available at https://lccn.loc.gov/2020051301

ISBN 978-1-61429-575-4   ebook ISBN 978-1-61429-599-0

25 24 23 22 21
5 4 3 2 1

Cover design by David Henry Lantz. Interior design by Tony Lulek. Set in Arno Pro 13/16.25.

Printed on acid-free paper that meets the guidelines for permanence and durability of the Production Guidelines for Book Longevity of the Council on Library Resources.

Printed in the United States of America.

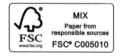

Please visit fscus.org.

To my family: Ed, Ben, Rebekah

Contents

Foreword by
His Holiness the Seventeenth Karmapa   ix

Introduction: Reading for Life   1

1. Reading Anew   11
2. Putting Down Anger: Uncovering Fear   19
3. Oriented by Love   41
4. Living with Uncertainty: When Will I Die?   63
5. Receiving Care   87
6. Grieving for and with Living Loved Ones   121
7. Companionship Follows Absence   149
8. "Not Dead Yet"   173

Acknowledgments and Thanks   181
Bibliography: Recommended Companions   185
Index   189
About the Author   195

Foreword

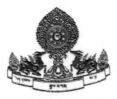

The Karmapa

I have known Karen Derris for much of the time that she has been living with her diagnosis of terminal brain cancer and have been witness to her work to find a way to orient herself by love rather than fear. I am confident that this orientation, which also serves as the basis of this book, will be beneficial not only to her but also to others who are living with terminal cancer and other illnesses.

All cultures have their own ways of living with the universal reality of death. Buddhist traditions encourage looking death in the eye and reflecting deeply on what is seen there. In our modern world, many cultures increasingly shy away from such clear-eyed seeing. It is clear that Professor Derris does not. In this time when a pandemic has made its way all over the planet, I believe this book could offer comfort and help to many people looking for guides to living aware of the reality of death all around us. To do so takes courage and compassion, and this book both displays and teaches both qualities.

As a Buddhist laywoman, an academic scholar, and university teacher of Buddhist literature, Professor Derris has found in Buddhist narratives friends to keep her company as she learns to live with her disease, and at the same time to live fully with the certainty of her mortality and the uncertainty of the time of her death. Karen shows us how various Buddhist stories—several of which she and I have discussed together—when encountered with an open, vulnerable heart, can transform every life experience into a way to live in service of others.

Seventeenth Karmapa, Ogyen Trinley Dorje

Introduction: Reading for Life

Instinctually, I turn to books as my first uncertain step into living with my brain cancer diagnosis. However, I am warned away from reading about my disease as it will, I'm told, throw me into states of terror and despair. I'm not interested in knowing the details of my cancer. Instead, I am searching for guides to help me process new experiences and those experiences still to come; aside from searching for books to read, nothing else about this is instinctual. I read memoirs by people who live with cancer, undergo treatment, and move closer to death.

I search for companions as I enter into a lonely new experience. Lonely, even though I am surrounded by loving family and friends, near and far, whose offers of every kind of help make me feel far from alone. The acute experience of the impermanence of my formerly healthy body now controlled by a terminal illness, my days consumed with prolonged medical treatment—it is impossible to fully share these things with those who haven't experienced some part of it themselves. I hear many well-meaning but clichéd truths: "We all could die at any time; a person could die from COVID or have a massive heart attack."

This is true, and we all probably know someone who died from the latter, if not from the former. The thing that I am experiencing that is different, living with a terminal illness, one without a cure, is that I live with the known source of my death already inside of my body. It creates an experience of being temporarily alive.

Much that I read in those cancer memoirs resonates deeply. I carry snippets, sentences, and images from these books around with me. They pop up into my conscious thought at times that don't always instantly make sense to me, but they do help me feel less alone. I gravitate toward women's memoirs (but not exclusively) and especially (but not only) toward memoirs by people who, like me, have careers as academics. All of these people integrate their living experiences of cancer with ideas and concepts that shape their minds, outlooks, and emotions.

These authors show me that while living with a terminal disease is new to me, I already have resources to draw upon, to help myself find a way to live well despite my increased awareness of the many ways my body—my brain, in particular—is changing. These authors drew from the ideas and questions to which they had dedicated their personal and professional lives—for how can practices of the mind be disentangled from the ways the rest of the body lives?

One of my newly found guides is a novelist, among others are a philosopher, a cultural critic, even a brain surgeon dying from brain cancer. Each of them found a deeply personal way to keep their footing as the ground of the familiar shifted this way and that, up and down, from treatments, declines, reprieves, and into the final steps of dying. In these memoirs I see a method I might employ for living with the traumatic certainty of my cancer diagnosis and the also-traumatic vagueness of prognosis and progression.

I read a handful of memoirs before; now they are surrounding me. When my nightstand can no longer hold them all, piles build up on the floor by my bedside. While I reach out to these memoirs, Buddhist narratives reach out to me. I don't have to search for them.

Stories from many Buddhist literary traditions take up many of my bookshelves in my office, my home, and more figuratively, in my mental library. They have accompanied me for years. I have dedicated my professional life to studying them. Reading and interpreting Buddhist narratives forms and reshapes my mind. They inspire the ways I intentionally aspire to live. These stories expand my understanding of what is real, and they show me the importance of imagination for measuring truth by its effectiveness for positive transformation on the axes of wisdom and compassion. In order to be a good reader, the mythical truths of these Buddhist stories are given as much weight as materialist, secular perspectives.

Now, I am reading these stories anew as I look for guides for living with my illness as a new, embodied experience of the foundational Buddhist teaching of impermanence.

These stories are of varying lengths and forms. Some grow from an image, a phrase, even just a word. Most I know from literary sources, but others are shaped by a visual narration of a story in a mural painting or a sculpture, strong images I can still see. Only a few have been told to me orally. Like most of you, I assume, I encounter stories as a reader. These stories invite us to participate with our imaginations and our own experiences. If we do so we might find ourselves stepping into the spaces they create for us. In turn, we can, if we wish, take these stories into us. We might tie a piece of a story to our own experience in order to reflect upon who we are and how we experience impermanence—today, tomorrow, years ago—through the guidance of a storied companion that speaks particularly to us.

The stories I will include here offer me this invitation and I accept it. I aim to read respectfully, gratefully, and humbly. I do not know everything about their literary traditions or their cultural or historical contexts. Fortunately, this is not my goal. I merely hope to share how the stories I retell here guide me through my own ever-transforming, acute experience of impermanence. I'm no longer observing impermanence from a distance; I'm crashing into it, or it into me.

The stories that naturally occur to me now are those I have known over time. These are stories I love. They are the narrative homes to the characters I love. The stories I retell are primarily from Theravada, Tibetan, and Jodo Shinshu traditions because these are the Buddhist traditions to which I have the deepest connections. My hope is that every reader will find these stories companionable. I also hope readers will use the methods of reading I share to engage their own imaginations with any story they wish to live inside, and with those stories they might wish to draw into themselves.

❧

The authors of the memoirs I read and the characters in Buddhist stories—some close to me in our shared time and some coming to me across great expanses of time and space—become companions, walking ahead of me through the terrain of terminal illness and approaching death. Sometimes, fear overcomes me. Especially as a new brain scan approaches—I need to hold the hand of someone by my side, someone who feels their body in ways that are similar to how I feel mine.

There is so much that is useful to me. A memoir, a newly encountered Buddhist story, even a letter. My husband, Ed, read me some lines from a letter printed in *The New Yorker* that the musician Leonard Cohen wrote to his former lover, Marianne, soon before her death:

> Well Marianne, it's come to this time when we are really so old and our bodies are falling apart and I think I will follow you very soon. Know that I am so close behind you that if you stretch out your hand, I think you can reach mine . . . I just want to wish you a very good journey. Goodbye old friend. Endless love, see you down the road.

Gillian Rose says in her memoir, *Love's Work*, "One story might do for many." The same is true here. Her book challenges me intellectually and emotionally to learn from my illness as a means for reflecting on how the work of love—the struggle to love and be loved—forms a full life, one that's imperfect but worth living until the end. She confronts her own terminal cancer as she asks why one friend lives with cancer almost the entirety of her ninety-six years, while another friend's body disintegrates from AIDS before his middle age. An obvious truth: death is a universal reality. Rose challenges me to feel this in-your-face experience of impermanence, to observe it, to learn from the reality of my body's illness.

Jenny Diski's defiant command that, after she dies, no one

better say that she bravely fought her cancer makes me laugh out loud. "Me too!" I say to myself. She recoiled at that cliché for her own reasons. For me, I detest its possible literal meaning that I am at war with my body. No! I refuse to recast myself into the role of warrior or victor in my own life. I'm not fighting on a battlefield that is my body. I am living. I am living with my cancer; it is a part of me. I feel no anger at my body, nor do I feel it is failing me. My cancer is a part of the transformation of my body. I would like the cancer cells to stop reproducing, to transform back into indolent, lazy cells (as my expert and humane oncologist Dr. Lai described them when they had been present but static for more than a decade). But I will not fight it; I will care for my body and experience its pain.

The treatments I have undergone these past years have all been intense. Some have pummeled my body; others cause ongoing pain. My body will not let me forget its impermanence. I can fantasize about a future time when my hair will be long again, living in Kyoto during my retirement, holding my first grandchild. But the neuropathic pain caused by the cancer and its treatment refocuses me away from these illusions and brings me back to the more likely reality that I will not be alive to actually experience any of those things.

I also laughed again at Jenny Diski's disbelief that she was going to write another "f'ing cancer memoir," but yes, that was what she did, and following behind her book *In Gratitude*, that is what I am doing too, in my own inexpert way. Reading Diski's work, I felt her courage and vulnerability, a need to make time meaningful. It allowed me to connect, even if she was wary of others interpreting or speaking for her experience. Her book inspires me to find the courage to be vulnerable too. In order to live my life fully, I need to allow other people's stories to help me find the courage to tell my own. I want to live a meaningful life; there's no time to waste on living a stupid one.

In my experience, reading narratives is a practice in cultivating imagination. It is impossible to make sense of a story without entering into a relationship with its characters, plot, and imagery. Imagination draws our senses into reading too.

What does it feel like to lay on the street where you are a spectacle of impermanence? How can boredom be tolerated when your body is bedridden? Is the duvet scratchy or smooth, warm or cool? Is there a stench emitted from a colostomy bag? How does the food shared from a nun's begging bowl taste to a starving woman? Is her mouth too dry to effortlessly swallow?

By drawing stories into her own body, a reader builds the bonds of empathy and strengthens the capacity to feel and understand her links of interconnectedness with others, no matter how far apart in that chain they might be.

"We are links in Amida's golden chain of love." I hear this for the first time at the funeral of Masatoshi Nagatomi, a foundational professor of Buddhist studies in North America and a Jodo Shinshu priest. It is an affirmation of interconnectedness, joining those of us now living with those whose lives we read about in stories; we're all linked together in the sphere of Amida Buddha's love. I have carried this testimony of faith with me ever since; it is a source of consolation and inspiration.

❧

I feel linked to the stories in the *Therigatha*, the poems by the first Buddhist nuns. When I return to teaching in 2014, a few months after my second craniotomy—and new terminal diagnosis—I read Charles Hallisey's beautiful translation of

it with my college students. A common line among many of
those ancient nuns' poems, "I approached the nun; she seems
like someone I can trust," weaves the nuns' individual poems
and voices together as companions in the nuns' Sangha. These
poems encourage me to hear their invitation to join them, and I
do so by holding their words and stories in my hands, head, and
heart. As I read their briefly told but deep and complex stories,
I make sense of my own experience from their vantage points.
For instance, I hear the nun Ambapali reflecting on her embodied impermanence:

> The hairs on my head were once curly, black, like the
>   color of bees, now because of old age
> They are like jute.
> It's just like the Buddha, the speaker of truth, said,
> Nothing different than that.

This is me, too. I'd thought that my hair was my best feature.
It was long, thick, chestnut colored. Now it is short, regrow-
ing coarsely from full brain radiation. When I read Ambapali's
poem now, I feel like she is saying to me, "I know, sister, I know."
And now, I know too! Noticing this kind of simple similarity
can remain superficial if it isn't developed. Practicing reading,
or reading as practice, strengthens these links to those who
reach out their hands to us through their stories.

There are many Buddhist stories to share. I've chosen stories
that I've lived with for a long time, and now I re-read them anew
as a terminally ill person.

I read a poem or story slowly, repeatedly. I read out loud with
my voice and in my head. I imagine the tone and resonance of
the words as they are spoken by different characters. I try to

listen for the emotion. I let the words sink in as I pay attention to their effect. I expand the meanings of words and phrases as I travel between them. By memorizing a verse or phrase, I carry the story around with me, calling it to mind whenever, wherever I need it.

To imagine a story or a character as a companion is to take it into myself in order to invite transformation. I find that when I live with a question—this is maybe more fully expressed as "living within a question"—everything becomes potentially useful. I'm living inside the question of how to live fully while feeling my body devolving toward death. I'm living inside the question of how I can orient myself toward that inevitable future with love rather than fear.

Who I am and who I am not: I am a student and practitioner of Buddhism and an academic teacher of Buddhist traditions. I am not a Dharma teacher. I have boundless gratitude for my own lama, His Holiness the Seventeenth Karmapa, Ogyen Trinley Dorje, and other Dharma teachers; my respect for them makes it essential that those who meet me through this book see me clearly as a disciple on the path, aspiring to share my experience of impermanence and knowledge of Buddhist narratives, not only from the analytical mind of the scholar but also from *citta*—the Sanskrit/Pali word for the heart-mind. I aspire to be of some benefit to you, as your imagined presence in my heart-mind benefits me now.

May any merit resulting from my work of writing this book and yours by reading it help alleviate the suffering of all beings.

1. Reading Anew

For people who do not grow up in a Buddhist culture, one of the first Buddhist stories they likely encounter is Prince Siddhartha's first journey outside his father's palace. This episode occurs in his final lifetime as a bodhisattva—the one in which he will attain awakening and become a buddha. This is a crucial event for his movement toward nirvana. It is also a narration of events that are extremely ordinary but rarely reflected upon. It is a story of a young man when he has his first sighting of the impermanence of bodies: an old body, a sick body, and a dead body.

At Siddhartha's birth, sages foretold his two possible futures to his father, King Suddhodana: If his son were to become aware of impermanence and the suffering it causes, he would leave the royal life to become the world's greatest spiritual leader. If he were shielded from suffering, he would become the world's greatest emperor. Wanting his son to carry forward the family lineage, King Suddhodana kept his son "imprisoned" in his beautiful palace. Not only was he kept from learning of the existence of suffering, he was also surrounded by every kind of pleasure, which anesthetized him to the discomforts of ordinary life moments

As he grows into manhood, Siddhartha asks to leave the palace to see the city. In some versions of this story—and there are many versions—*devas*, celestial beings, plant the idea in the prince's thoughts. Without this first of many interventions by the devas, he might have remained blissed out on pleasure, never reaching the final stages of becoming a buddha. The devas know the prince must see forms of impermanence and suffering and reflect upon their causes if he is to find his path to nirvana.

With the devas' prodding, Prince Siddhartha makes it impossible for his father to prevent him from leaving the palace grounds; in some versions he sneaks out of the palace with the direct intervention of the gods. But in acquiescing to his son's trips outside, Suddhodana doesn't give up on his years of shielding Siddhartha from suffering; he merely shifts tactics. The king orders his city cleaned and decorated. In order to hide all signs of suffering, he commands that all the old, sick, and dead people in the city should be hidden away where his son will not be able to see them.

As this story is told in the *Buddhacharita*, a Sanskrit biography of the Buddha, when Prince Siddhartha leaves the palace, the procession route is bursting with healthy people, flowers, and banners, precisely as the king commands. In verse after verse the poet describes beautiful women leaning over their balcony railings, trying to catch their first sight of the prince. These descriptions of beauty effectively swallow up the few verses that describe the three forms of impermanent bodies that the prince does manage to glimpse over the course of three trips, effectively replicating the king's goal of hiding them. Like the Bodhisattva, we have to be attentive readers in order to stay focused on the presence of these particular bodies, the old man, the sick man, and the corpse.

There is so much going on in this scene of the Buddha's story; I feel like I could step into it. If I had first joined the throngs along the procession hoping to catch sight of the prince, my cancer-stricken body would probably feel off balance and in danger of falling. Perhaps I might find a spot to sit along the procession route—but then the king's men would pick up my sick body and deposit me in an alleyway, making sure I'm out of sight. But the devas wouldn't leave me there. In this existential tug of war, they would lift me up and return me to the procession route; they know that the Bodhisattva has to see the suffering caused by impermanence. Why would seeing my sick body be so powerful to cause this existential tug of war?

On the Bodhisattva's path, despite the efforts of his father, he still sees the old person, the sick person, and the dead person. He tunes out the enchanting noise of women's tinkling jewelry to hear the sick person crying out. He sees the old person stumbling as the crowd shoves her this way and that. He sees the dead body carried in its procession to the funeral grounds.

Seeing each of these forms of suffering shocks and disturbs the prince. "Will this happen to me too?" he asks his companion and chariot driver, Channa.

"Yes," is Channa's straightforward and deeply true response.

I wonder whether we could generate a similar existential bolt if we shifted the focus of the story from Siddhartha's point of view to those of the old, the ill, or the dying person? For people whose impermanence is pronouncedly embodied, what would they say to Siddhartha beyond "Yes, this happens to all people"? If it were me in that crowd, I'd say, "This is happening to me right now! Most people don't acknowledge their own impermanence. I *feel* my own impermanence!"

This scene from the Buddha's life has been depicted in many Buddhist artistic traditions. The painting that I see in my mind's eye is on a central pillar of a *vihara*—main hall—at the royal temple of Wat Suthat in Bangkok. Every surface of the hall is painted with narratives of the Buddha's previous lifetimes as the Bodhisattva, including this final one.

In the mural, beneath a flying deva's guiding presence, Prince Siddhartha is shown in his chariot moving through the city. There they are, the old, sick, and dead bodies. Channa drives the chariot, looking determinedly forward, eager to get the prince back to the curated experiences within the palace.

In stark contrast, the prince's head strains over his shoulder to keep these three suffering people in view for as long as possible. Each figure in the narrative mural is miniature but detailed. The old person, bent at the waist, could be saying, "I've so much farther to walk, where is my cane?" The sick person's head is thrown back, mouth open, gasping in agony, as though crying out, "Mother!" The dead body is represented as a skeleton outlined in black.

This tiny scene is one small part of the total path to awakening, but seeing it is the crucial event that helps the Bodhisattva realize the reality of impermanence and the suffering it causes.

Statues from across the Buddhist world depict Prince Siddhartha in what is called the "pondering pose," reflecting on the reality he encountered outside the palace walls. He sits with his crowned head bowed, one arm resting on a crossed leg, his hand on one of his cheeks. The posture is always lifelike, no matter the details of the particular statue. His body folds inward, supporting itself under the weight of his head and the burden of his crown. He sees nothing now but what his downward glance affords. He is, I imagine, replaying the sight of those impermanent bodies.

Even as Suddhodana sees his son in this state of despondency, he still doesn't give up. He tells the prince's friends to take him to a pleasure garden for another dose of sensual delight, but Siddhartha now refuses to eat the beautiful feasts or interact with the gorgeous, seductive women. The only thing he sees and willingly takes in is the fourth sign, a renunciant, who he saw on his last trip outside the palace.

This is another kind of body. Such a person willingly and deliberately changes their body by shaving their head, removing jewels, and wearing only robes sewn from rags. They move through the world in a different way and for a different purpose. Seeing this body inspires the Bodhisattva to find a path to alleviate the willful ignorance of impermanence and the suffering it causes.

Seeing just these four kinds of bodies changed the Bodhisattva's life completely. Is my sick body also that dangerous or powerful? On our first read, we might find this story impossible to believe, but we can use our own experiences as a foundation to begin to see how material reality intertwines with imagined reality in this story—as they do in much of Buddhist literature. In the narrative worlds, something need not be real to be true. While it may seem as though Siddhartha lives in a Sleeping Beauty–like castle, and it may feel impossible to relate his seemingly simple experience to our chaotic lives, connections are plentiful. Think of how parents shield their children from violent images on the television or turn off stories that describe war or famine. Alternately, once parents stop sheltering their children, many of them grow up on visual diets of death and destruction through video games and movies; this too can desensitize people from direct visual encounters with suffering and death.

Many of us cross the street rather than walk by the body of a homeless person. How many times have I found myself silently saying, "I just can't look"? Many of us look away from the disabled too.

Prince Siddhartha, our Buddha, saw those who were feeling the embodiment of their impermanence. He held them with his gaze. For those of us who are feeling impermanence eroding our selves, being seen can feel like being held. His focused gaze, his embrace, is so accepting; he places himself in the position of the sick person, aged person, and dying person. "Will this happen to me too?" In my new acute experience of illness, others' willingness to see my embodied suffering, and my efforts to see others, feels like an ethical, healing act.

⸎

Soon after my first diagnosis of a not-yet-terminal stage of this cancer, I stopped dyeing my hair. I had been coloring my gray hair brown for years; for all those years with my college students I felt like a hypocrite every time I discussed the ways people resist the evidence of impermanence and failed to admit that I was one of the resisters. Dyeing my gray hair was a way to hide the signs of my aging process, a refusal to accept it. That first craniotomy in 2014 put an end to that resistance. How could I continue to put chemicals on my scalp knowing what I know of the cancerous cells in my brain?

As my gray and white hair grew in, the signs of my aging sometimes made me, or who I am, invisible. Checking in for my kids' biannual dental appointment, I'm innocently asked by the smiling receptionist who I am. "The kids' grandmother?"

I want to shout, "Their grandmother!?" (Or maybe I did shout, much to my kids' embarrassment.) She's known me for years, and besides I am only in my mid-forties! Other than the color of my hair, nothing else had changed about my appearance. Was my white hair some sort of invisibility cap? Viewed as an older woman, I seem a little hard to see, not because I'm actually invisible, but because I am accepting my changing, aging self, and that is challenging to make sense of in our youth-obsessed culture. It takes me some time to settle into it too, as I realize by my enraged overreaction. With time, my white hair helps me feel authentic in my body. Rather than holding on to the brown color of my youth, my curls of white hair look something like a beautiful little puffed cloud drifting along with me as I move.

The presence of my cancer is less visible than signs of aging. My chemo drug didn't make all of my hair fall out, but I cut it short to even out the shaved area from the craniotomies and the bits that have fallen out from my radiation treatment.

I want people to know that my body is changing, but it isn't obvious to see; it is hard for many people to hear when I do have the courage to talk about my situation. I want to tell my own story, I am lonely, and I want people to know what I am going through—but I hesitate. I destroy the fun at several dinner gatherings by answering someone's question of why I'd cut my hair with a short explanation that I'd had full brain radiation.

Sometimes I feel like I am being cruel by honestly answering a simple question: "You look great! How are you?" "Not so good...I have brain cancer." People tear up, retreat into corners, ignore me for months.

Maybe, like Prince Siddhartha, being confronted by my

cancerous body led to an experience of existential shock for friends and acquaintances too. Maybe, like him, they wonder, "This happened to Karen. Could this happen to me too?"

During a two-year period of intensive treatment, I regularly see the tumor in my brain on my bimonthly MRI scan. "It's all in my head"—really. I think of my brain as my mind: the source of my delight in thinking, learning, interpreting. It never really occurs to me, even now, that it is an organ with mutating cells and tissue that is healthy or unhealthy. These MRIs are my window into seeing my brain as it changes. My doctors are looking for evidence of impermanence.

Hearing that I had a brain tumor was my existential crisis. I remember pleading, beginning to cry, with the oncologist who gave us the results of my very first MRI scan: "But I have a one-year-old child!" As if that had anything to do with it. As if just that truth should change the MRI and render the tumor invisible and unknown again. How could this be happening? It is happening. Eighteen years later, it still is. Dying has come much closer now since my diagnosis of grade IV brain cancer, glioblastoma. All cancers are destructive. This one can be, and usually is, a monster.

2. Putting Down Anger: Uncovering Fear

When I am thirteen years old my mother was killed in a car crash as she drove me to school. I survive; she died instantly. She had a bad death. She knew it was coming only in the terrifying split second before it happened. No time to prepare her mind, to tend to the connections that had formed her life, no goodbyes. I can still see her shocked face in my peripheral view as our car was about to crash head-on into the oncoming vehicle. I hear her scream as I lose consciousness in that same second.

Surviving the car accident that killed my mother brought every clichéd lesson of the fragility and the unpredictability of life to the fore: every day is precious, live it like there's no tomorrow, we never know how much time we'll have. These sayings are too superficial to provide real guidance for living. The mundane repetitions of living one day into the next are real. The right lesson, it seems to me, is to make visible the meaning of those mundane repetitions, but I didn't know that at thirteen years of age.

Nor did I know it at age four. That was how old I am when I first realize that my life will end. Maybe this seems young, or abnormal—but it wasn't an encounter with death I'm attempting to trace to its originating point; it is the first time that I knew I myself will die. Bizarrely, knowing I will die precedes my awareness that I am alive. I have just one or two photos to generate visual memories of the event, and there are pieces of the story that no one told me until I was fully grown, yet I still remember details no one else witnessed.

My mom is cleaning in the family room while my dad's visiting mom and stepfather nap upstairs. I want to help my mom with her cleaning, but of course I wasn't helpful: I slow her down, I intrude upon the private space she must have sought. The joy I find in a spray bottle that afternoon is something I would re-encounter decades later with my own kids.

My joy is unshared and short-lived on that day. I can clearly see myself standing in front of the television catching the rivulets of cleaning fluid racing my rag down the side. I don't know if I saw her in the reflection of the screen, coming up behind me with a raised glass bottle, before she struck me on the back of my head.

Next, I'm on my grandma's lap in the front seat of the car. I clearly remember looking at my mom from the corner of my eye as she drove us to the hospital. Her face looked stone cold, focused, removed. My grandma held a dishtowel tightly to the back of my head. It must have saturated quickly with blood. I clearly remember whispering in her ear, "Don't let me die, Grandma, I don't want to die." Somehow, I knew then that at some point I would no longer be alive, and I also knew that I didn't want to not be.

I did repeatedly whisper these words into my grandma's ear. My dad's sister, my beloved aunt Joan, confirmed this for me years later. My grandma had died before I began to ask questions and put together a more complete understanding of what happened that day, one beyond what my memories tell me. But as soon as Grandma returned home to New York she replayed the scene for her daughter, Aunt Joan. I said it over and over while I sat on her lap in the front seat while my mother drove us to the hospital. Some of my blood got onto her dress; the kitchen towels were totally saturated with it.

My sweet grandma. She was my primary source of unconditional love in my childhood. She always called me her "baby doll." I am the youngest of her grandchildren. She called all four of her granddaughters "doll girl," but as her youngest, my grandma called me "baby doll." Aunt Joan still calls me "doll girl," and now my daughter is "doll girl" too.

When my dad was seventeen, his father died from a heart attack, after a life of long days selling vegetables at wholesale markets in New York City. An Ellis Island Jew, half of his siblings had changed their name. His wife, my grandma, must have felt lost when visiting the WASP-y Boston suburb where my parents first settled, with its newly built synagogue and neighborhoods of stately homes sustained by wealth that had been passed on for generations. Neighborhoods like the one we lived in had only recently started selling homes to Jews. Her daughter-in-law cracked open her own little girl's head while she napped upstairs? What *mishigas* (Yiddish for "craziness") is this?

There was no way to understand the misdirection of my mother's out-of-control rage. I didn't—couldn't—understand it either. I carried that heavy confusion with me as I grew up, and I sometimes brought that early life experience into the new ideas and the new stories I encountered in my studies. Although I didn't immediately see my mom in the character of Milarepa's mother, as I continued to re-read this story, I found myself making those connections.

When I first studied *The Life of Milarepa* as a work of literature and ethics, I did not yet see a way to view his mother with compassion. I only saw her as a source of harm. Milarepa, an eleventh-century Tibetan saint, was born into a wealthy family. After the death of his father, his uncle and aunt stole his patrimony and made him, his mother, and sister live in poverty, attending on them as servants. Milarepa's mother seethed with rage and used Milarepa as the instrument for violent revenge; she forced her son to learn black magic in order to kill his aunt and uncle's family. Where Milarepa's mother's actions were a methodical—if rage-filled—response to injustice, my mom's act of abuse erupted from an untreated mental illness, and I imagine it was stress that lit it on fire in any given moment.

My analytical mind must take many steps to begin to read with empathy. When I reflect upon the many times I've re-read the life of Milaepa, I recall that with empathy and compassion is the very first way it is read to me. I am nineteen years old, living with a Tibetan family on the outskirts of Kathmandu as a part of a study-abroad program in 1989. The mother of that family is nurturing and loving. I am like a baby: I speak only a few phrases of Tibetan, and I don't know how to do nearly anything. "Ama-la," or "mother," as I'm told to call her, washes all my clothes and uses a graphic version of the Milarepa story to educate me in this classic of Tibetan Buddhism. For hours, she would sit on her couch with me teaching me the story by pointing to pictures and sharing her emotional responses to nearly every scene. She cried hardest for Milarepa's mom: for the loss of her husband, the harm inflicted upon her by her in-laws, and her separation from her son, Milarepa. She read with so much emotion.

Years later, now as a professor of religious studies, I ask my college students to imagine a context in our own time and place that could help us not only understand the conditions that led Milarepa's mother to act the way she did, but also to give rise to feelings of empathy for her.

What if, I ask my students at the beginning of an exercise in cultivating a reader's imagination, Milarepa's widowed mother had become homeless after her husband's family forged a check and stole all their money? What if her daughter became sick, and since she could afford neither medicine nor a doctor, she gets so desperate that she sends her son, Milarepa, to steal some over-the-counter drugs. Of course, he gets caught and tells the police that his mom made him do it, and as a result both her children get taken away by child protection services. It's not so difficult, with small narrative adjustments, to make this story make sense in our time.

After years of distress and poverty, Milarepa's mother wanted more than the return of their rightful property. She wanted compensation, with interest, for their harm and suffering. The violence she unleashed, pushing her son to kill dozens of in-laws, is illustrative; we can relate to that level of rage and desire for vengeance, even if the details of the ancient story aren't easy to completely reconcile to our modern worldview. And yet, we can ask of both Milarepa's mother and my own: what brings a mother to harm children? Reading for living invites us to jump back and forth between narrative frames, the ones we reflect upon in our own experiences and the ones we read in texts, between Milarepa's mother's acts of revenge and my mother's psychic explosion.

Milarepa kills dozens of people in fear that his mother will harm herself. In remorse, he seeks out a Buddhist teacher, Marpa, who then guides him to enlightenment. In a darkly ironic way, Milarepa's mother's violence was a catalyst for his liberation, as difficult as that might be to accept.

Entering in my own way into this narrative of trauma and recovery, I am the child harmed by her mother. I see myself lying on a surgical table beneath a tent of surgical clothes, nurses in front of me as the doctor stitches up my scalp. "Stay still, please don't move." I've heard this instruction in my brain cancer treatment so many times in recent years that I can't be sure if it's what I remember or what I assume they said. It doesn't matter. Little me, struck with a glass bottle by my own mother, stayed still. Maybe this is when my determination to be a perfect patient formed. If I behave perfectly, maybe I will not be hurt even more. What else would they have said? I don't remember. I hope they would have said, "How could a mother do this? This poor child."

My mother was a complicated woman. Like Milarepa's mother, she had been harmed by others. She suffered from mental illness that was never properly treated. She felt every emotion passionately. I loved her intensely. I have a few pictures of me from that time. White gauze winds around my head, mummy-style. In one photo, I stand by my mom's side as she sits on our lawn, both of us reaching the same height. My arm rests around her shoulder. I look sad; my mother has a forced smile. Is it possible that I felt compassion for her in that moment? She was my mother; I loved her with a child's uncomplicated heart. She was my mother; she harmed me because of conditions I didn't know or understand.

My maternal grandmother abused my mother, mentally and

physically. I don't know many details. When I was grown, my father told me that my grandmother had frequently threatened suicide. She would tell my mother, "When you get home from school, you'll find my dead body in the oven." How did my mom walk to school with her mother's voice in her head without imagining her mother's head in the oven? Did she tune it out? Train herself not to hear it? Or maybe the feeling of danger as something that was beyond her control settled deep into her psyche. From that view, she was brought up to be out of control.

My own mother didn't threaten. She acted out. And those actions were out of control. I don't believe any of her harmful actions were planned or calculated, and for some reason this makes it easier to forgive her. But only after many years of emotional excavation, first through therapy and then working with new perspectives of interconnectedness that I learned through Dharma teachings, could I face and overcome my anger.

How far back did those cycles of abuse go? Did my great-grandmother, Grandma Annie, carry them with her from Poland alongside the challah bread bowl that now sits in my kitchen cupboard? How are the cycles stopped? What would be the intervention preventing them from rolling into the present and on into the future? It is too simple to assert, as I once sternly told myself, that I will resolve to make self-control the essential quality of my parenting. Of course, there is much more to it than a decision made with a critical mind. Self-control also arises by feeling compassion for those who lack it, caught up in a dangerous whirlpool of causation.

The Sinhala (the language of Sri Lankan Buddhists) story "The Demoness Kali" helps me reframe my reflections of my mother. This story reels between two women whose fear of one another, and the rage they hurl at each other, grows into a murderous vengeance that is taken out on each other's children across lifetime after lifetime.

It all begins with the all-too-human problems of fear and jealousy. A young wife is barren, and a second wife is brought into the household to produce an heir. The first wife, acting out of her fear for her position in the family, makes the second wife miscarry each of her pregnancies. The second wife, bereft of her children, vows to be reborn in forms that will enable her to kill any children the first wife gives birth to in any of her future lives.

The vow begets generations of violence. If one is born as a hen, the other is born as a cat who eats the hen's chicks; a fawn is eaten by a tigress. On and on the enmity and harm spins. Bound together in lifetime after lifetime in whatever bodies they take, human or animal, the reincarnation of the vengeful second wife kills the other's children.

Finally, the Buddha's intervention brings this cycle of murderous revenge to a stop. The first wife is reborn as a human being, and the second wife as a demoness. Thinking that the only way to protect her child from the demoness is to gain the protection of the Buddha, the mother runs to him and lays her child at his feet. The Buddha offers the mother and child shelter, but he also teaches her that in order to truly save her child, she must break the cycle of violence. She must shift her perspective from fear and anger to forgiveness and compassion.

By explaining to the woman the origin of the violence, the Buddha gives her some of the tools she needs to end it. She could now understand the history she shared with the demoness, how over lifetimes they attacked each other in anger and vengeance. But this intellectual understanding of the situation is not enough; only compassion would calm the whirlpool. By understanding their shared history and generating compassion for the demoness, by forgiving herself her own vile act that initiated the vicious cycle, and forgiving the demoness all her subsequent acts of revenge, the mother could overcome her anger and fear. The Buddha instructs the woman to let go of her fear of the demoness and trust her; he tells her to place her child in the demoness's arms.

Like the woman in this story I could choose to feel compassion for my mother and to free myself from my rage. To break the cycle of abuse is a choice, a choice I make from a position of love—not the discriminating, calculating mind that says, "My mother was bad, she abused me; I am good, I do not hurt my children." I can intellectually understand the causes of my mother's behavior, but I cannot forgive her unless I can empathize with her, until I can feel safe placing my children in her arms. This is not easy.

❦

Forty-one years after my mother bashed my head with a bottle, I'm again lying in a hospital bed, my head in white gauze following my first craniotomy, which removed 90% of a cancerous tumor from the back of my right frontal lobe. I ask my husband, Ed, to take a picture of me holding the teddy bear our daughter, Rebekah, had sent to the hospital with me. I keep my prayer beads, blessed by His Holiness the Seventeenth Karmapa, wrapped around the bear so I won't lose them in the bed with its many cables attaching me to monitoring machines.

We record small moments for reasons we don't know in that moment. I wanted a picture. Perhaps, like the pictures I have with my bandaged head beside my mother, I have an instinctual confidence that it will later provide a vantage point—gained by distance in time, other experiences, or new worldviews—through which I will be able make sense of all of these experiences.

Looking back at those photos of little-me with a bandaged head, I see my arm around my mother's shoulders, standing by her side as she sat on the lawn. I look somber, concerned, for myself, but for her too. From my childhood memories I remember her as beautiful, playful, a dear friend to many, and sometimes out of control. Her lack of control stayed with her right up to the second she died. In the moments before her death, she must have been flung about within the car as it flipped upside down onto its roof, finally coming to a stop against a fence at the bottom of a small hill on the side of the two-lane country road.

As I regain consciousness in that car, my plan for this scenario quickly comes into focus. As a child of an abusive mother, I developed strategies for surviving every possibility of chaos and harm she might conjure. This is how I live with the impermanence of life wrought by my mother; I prepared myself for every possible way she might kill me. My plan for the car-crash scenario, crafted one evening during a particularly erratic drive home, somewhat naively had me getting out of the car and finding help.

As it turned out, it isn't easy to get out of the car. I am pinned under my mother's body. When I manage to crawl out from under her and through the open driver-side window, help is already there. Many cars had pulled over and drivers had rushed down the slope. Their goal is to get me away from the car and from my mom's dead body. A young man walks me up the small hill, across the road, and we sit in the grass. He begins to pray. "Dear Lord. Please save this girl's mommy." He prays to Jesus too. I tell him we are Jewish, but I guess it is OK. When the ambulance arrives, the driver puts me and the people from the other car into the back. I wonder where my mom is. The ambulance driver tells me sternly, "Your mom's dead. Do *not* get hysterical."

It really did happen just like this. I still can't believe he spoke to me this way. It becomes another traumatic dimension of the whole horrific event. Would asking questions have qualified as hysterical? I didn't ask any until we got to the hospital and I saw one of our neighbors, a doctor, while being wheeled into the ER. "Can you call my dad, please? He'll be at his office."

As you would expect, traumatic experiences continue to unfold over the next hours and days. When my father arrives, his face shows that he too is in shock. He finds me in a hospital bed with my long hair knotting into a blood-soaked mat of my own and my mother's blood mingled with glass, dirt, and rocks. The doctors fear that I have some internal injury and instruct me to lie still. Always, the doctors are telling me to lie still.

My body was not seriously hurt, although decades later I wonder if the blow to my head in that accident damaged my brain in a way that led to my cancer. My oncologist says studies don't back up that theory, and as the Buddha himself taught, the origins of suffering aren't relevant; our whole focus needs to be on removing the present cause of suffering. When I disclosed my speculations to Charlie Hallisey, my former dissertation advisor and now lifelong friend and teacher, he looked at me from the corner of his eye and said with great empathy, "It's all too over-determined." Charlie is one of my closest companions through all of this. He is a brilliant scholar and teacher of Theravada literature. Ed and I met at Harvard in his Buddhist ethics course; five or six years later he performed our wedding ceremony.

As the narrator of my life story in this book, I separate the two: I am author and I am subject. I reflect upon my life from an imagined distance. I survived childhood abuse, a traumatic accident, and I am now surviving the ongoing trauma of living with a terminal brain tumor. There is space, temporally and emotionally, between traumatic events, and between the observer and the observed. I must keep those spaces. If I do, I can find a perspective that even trauma of these sorts do change with time. Experiences too are impermanent, and they can transform toward healing.

As I grew older, it became harder for me to keep all of my mother's complex, contradictory qualities in my picture of her. As the range of my memories faded, the range of my emotions narrowed as well. Because of this thinning, my rage toward her grew. The process that led me to fully know that I deserve care without harm meant identifying and clearly seeing my mother as my abuser. For many years this was all I could see, and my fear of her led me to doubt myself. I came to wonder if I should have children at all. I had to ask, will I hurt my children, as my mother had hurt my sister and me, and my mother's mother had hurt her?

⌒⌘⌒

In my first year of graduate school at Harvard Divinity School, I encountered the teachings of the Tibetan monk-scholar Tsongkhapa in Charlie Hallisey's course on Buddhist ethics. We were working with Tsongkhapa's idea that over our countless numbers of lifetimes all beings had at one time or another been our mother.

Taking this theoretical perspective into daily life we can see every being we encounter as having been our mother at least once, if not more times. And, because our mothers have cared for us in ways that allowed us to flourish, we must reciprocate that care now to every being—as if they were our mother.

Soon after reading of this practice, "The Sevenfold Cause and Effect," and interested in using it to generate *bodhichitta*—the mind of compassion—I stand in the doorway of Charlie's office and ask, "What if we didn't have a mother who cared for us in a way that allowed us to flourish? What if our mother caused us harm?"

I am ashamed to ask these questions. It feels shameful to be an abused child; just as now I sometimes feel ashamed to have brain cancer. It doesn't make sense, but I feel the shame. In that initial exchange, Charlie didn't look away, as he might have had he been irritated or embarrassed by my questions. He replied, "One way that every mother does care for her child is the act of carrying them in her womb so that the child can be born. Even those months are the basis for a universal ethic of reciprocity."

I think I felt it at the time, but certainly now, after all the decades of our friendship, I know that Charlie saw through the hypothetical phrasing of my questions while also respecting the distance I needed to be able to connect my life experience to Tsongkhapa's teaching. As I reflect upon it now, this is one of many similarly short instances when I learn to read for living.

The story of the monk Angulimala and the commentary on it by His Holiness the Seventeenth Karmapa also helped me see my mother in all her complexity, to meet her anew and to once again feel my love for her.

Angulimala was a dutiful brahmin son who studied under a Vedic pandit, becoming the head student and loyally following his teacher's commands. The story begins when Angulimala is falsely accused of making romantic advances toward the teacher's wife. Spurred on by his baseless jealousy, the teacher commands Angulimala to make a necklace of one thousand fingers, each from a different person, thereby driving him to become a horrific serial killer, the details of which are drawn out in voyeuristic gore.

When Angulimala's necklace needs only one more finger, he searches out a final victim. By now, everyone knows to hide from the man garlanded in bloody fingers, but his mother, longing for him to stop his murderous madness, places herself in his path. She understands that sacrificing herself will end her son's suffering and also save the life of his next victim. But before Angulimala can reach her, the Buddha places himself between them, appearing to offer himself as Angulimala's final victim. Yet no matter how he tries, Angulimala cannot lay his hands on the Buddha; whenever he comes close, the Buddha appears to be moving away, only stopping when Angulimala himself halts. After Angulimala expresses his frustration over the chase, the Buddha states, "I have stopped, when will you?" He then commands Angulimala: "Stop!" The power of the Buddha's word is all that it takes to bring Angulimala's mind to equanimity and to cease his murderous rampage. The Buddha ordains him, and Angulimala goes on to attain awakening.

I find this story difficult to hold in my mind. Its fantastical and gory elements make it beyond distasteful and unbelievable: it is an obvious allegory—the name "Angulimala" means "garland of fingers." Yet with just a few imaginative steps I can think of plenty of examples of this scale of killing in our times. It is the psychological treatment and transformation that are harder to bring close: without a buddha's command, how does a person gain control of their seemingly uncontrollable mind? Perhaps, most puzzling of all, how does the Buddha so easily embrace a serial killer and give him a new exalted life in the Sangha? How could such a person be redeemed?

The Karmapa's commentary on this story focuses on the conditions that lead Angulimala to his destructive behavior. He wasn't a monster by nature: conditions had transformed him into a person who performed monstrous deeds. Just as those conditions outside of himself led to his sociopathic actions, different conditions could transform him again into a disciple and then a practitioner of compassion. In Sri Lanka he is seen as a protector of pregnant and new mothers.

In his reading of this story, the Karmapa asks us to question if our distaste should be directed at Angulimala, or his teacher who ordered him onto this horrific path, or the teacher's wife who caused the jealousy, or the unknown encounters that had spurred her attention to Angulimala, or . . . , or . . . I've come to read Milarepa's mother in a similar way: is she to be blamed for the violence Milarepa committed, or the uncle and aunt who drove her to seek revenge, or the husband who died, or . . . , or . . .

My anger at my mother arose from the condition of being seriously hurt by the person from whom I deserved care and protection. She was instead a source of terror and pain. But should my anger be directed at my mother, or her mother who had done the same to her, or the inadequate mental health care that hadn't helped my mother learn self-control? Or . . . Or . . .?

By destabilizing the target for my anger, I finally saw that there was no target. If the target of my anger could dissipate, so too could my anger and reveal what it hid.

When I was still quite young, maybe five or six, I would walk in tight, fast circles repeating the phrase "k/not in my stomach."

I don't know if I meant "not in my stomach," as in, "don't hit me there," or "knot in my stomach," as in, "my fear had grown into a mass that kept me spinning." My mother often screamed at my sister and me, pulling our hair while brushing it so tightly we'd cry, and hit us with wooden spoons. In her calm playful times, she would send us into giggles with tickle fits. But when she lifted me up at age four or five, saying, "You are so sweet I'm going to cook you up for my dinner," I believed she'd do it. In my early forties my internal anger and fear still sat inside me equivalent to a physical mass; it was up to me to loosen my grip and put it down.

After spending so many years trying to bring the sources of my anger into focus, the Karmapa's teachings led me to broaden my perspective. Anger covers a deeper emotion: fear. Anger was protective armor for a scary life. Once I got down to the fear, I could hold it, like a cradled child. It was only then that I could finally put the anger down.

Kisa Gotami, a nun whose story is told in a poem of the *Therigatha*, guided me through this process of putting down my anger. She is famed in the Theravada narrative tradition as one of the earliest nuns. Her story is usually read as a figure epitomizing what grief can become when the reality of impermanence is rejected. She is introduced as a young mother whose child has just died. Refusing to release her son's body for funeral rituals, Kisa Gotami carries his dead body through her village desperately looking for anyone who might be able to bring him back to life. When she encounters the Buddha, he tells her he can do what she asks only if she brings him a mustard seed—a staple item in any Indian kitchen—from a family that has not known death.

Hopefully, and then desperately, she knocks on doors asking

her question, "Has anyone in your family died?" all the while holding her dead child. She is unable to find such a mustard seed. These encounters shift her perspective on the request she made to the Buddha and his directive to her. Every family knows death. She is not alone in her grief. Just as these people have survived it, so too could she. Returning to the Buddha without a mustard seed but with a mind developing equanimity, she is ready to put down her son's dead body.

Kisa Gotami's act is one of forming a connection to others who have also experienced intimate encounters with impermanence. I love that the Buddha does not tell her what to do; he does not give her an abstract teaching on the reality she refused to see. He guides her through a process that enables her to come to this new understanding and emotional state for herself.

Kisa Gotami's story is usually interpreted as portraying the power of the grief that arises when we resist the reality of impermanence and death. What could be more horrific than the death of one's child? Kisa Gotami is desperate for some magic to reverse the course of impermanence. We should feel empathy and grieve alongside her at the death of her child.

For me, Kisa Gotami can also be interpreted as a woman who is holding on to an identity that she no longer should: that of mother. As that role is dependent on the life of her son, upon his death she no longer has the condition that determined that status. It is not difficult to imagine why she would cling to the role. She was a young woman whose life in her in-laws' house was probably harsh and oppressive, as was the norm in pre-modern India (and is not so different even today). I imagine too that she may have felt anger for a role she might have been forced into, and for an evaluation of her worth that was only alleviated by the birth of a son.

When that son died, her grief was likely mingled with questions of what would happen to her next. Her searching for the mustard seed could also be read as a searching for a liberating space outside of the ones she knew in the domestic sphere as daughter, wife, mother, and daughter-in-law. She would find that space within the nuns' Sangha.

Clinging to emotions can fix us into roles that we otherwise would outgrow; grieving mother, abused daughter. As Kisa Gotami learned to put down her grief, her story inspired me to put down my anger, an emotion I clung to much like she had clung to her son's dead body. My anger made me feel protected in my dangerous early life, but the time had come to uncover my fear and move on and fully embrace my life as professor, mother, and wife, and I could only do that by putting down that anger.

Living with Kisa Gotami's story, I sometimes catch sight of her and follow her as she guides me through this process of putting down my anger. I can almost feel her hand reaching back for mine. Putting down anger has been a crucial step to experience my own impermanence as a journey deeper into love rather than its loss.

⌘

When Ben was two and a half my husband and I had to rush him to the emergency room. I remember him screaming in pain as one doctor after another examined his left leg, badly broken from a playground accident.

The first doctor at urgent care had awkwardly commented, "You are obviously good parents. He's clearly well cared for." "Yes . . .?" I replied. To my husband: "Why do they keep asking us the same questions?" I'm confused, looking pleadingly into my husband's eyes. Our connection can be very strong, allowing us to communicate rapidly and with few words. "They think we did it," he tells me. "They think we broke his leg." I have no idea that children's broken femurs are often the result of abuse. Ed calmly answers a hospital staff member's question again with a factual description. "We were at the playground, he slipped off the swing, maybe two feet. It was my fault, I took my hand off his back, for just a second." Ed is steely cool when he tells the next resident to keep his hands away from our beautiful little boy unless he is going to do something to ease his pain.

Ben's eyes are just as blue as my mom's. For the first time they are full of fear and pain. Once he's been admitted to the hospital, the ward nurse asks us the same series of questions and then signs off on the child protection form: no further investigation needed.

Connecting closely to my childhood experiences, I'm shaking. I tell Ed, "I'm glad they asked, I'm glad so many people asked. Thank god, they check, of course they need to ask . . ." It is so deeply painful for me to be suspected of child abuse, even as I can see how important it is for such a rigorous screening protocol.

Even in the chaotic, shocking moments in the pediatric emergency room my mind goes back to when I was the child—with a broken skull rather than leg, and with a mother who had done it. My husband purposefully directed any possible blame—although there was none—to himself. He shielded me from the trauma any blame toward me would unleash.

After days of his little legs suspended in traction, Ben's body was enclosed in a cast from his chest to his feet. Over the next six weeks I wash Ben's half-body cast, blow it dry, rub baby powder and baking powder into it—anything in order to keep it clean. It is no easy task with its cut-out for the diaper and Ben's body inside still bursting with activity. Resilient, he drags himself on his elbows to play with his toys and to get around his pre-school classroom.

His loving teachers lift his inflexible body from a rented wheelchair. We call his cast a turtle shell, in an attempt to keep as much of his discomfort light and undramatic as possible. He runs his Matchbox cars over it, designating parts of his cast as ramps, freeways, and parking garages.

"Wow, you kept it so clean," a nurse approvingly compliments me at an orthopedic checkup. "That must have been hard. I don't think I've ever seen a cast this clean after six weeks." I had taken the task as a test of my fitness as a mother, and beyond that as a test that I would not be my mother. I pass, but fear flipped my reality; in my upside-down world I was convinced that should I fail as a mother, I would be exposed to the world as my mother. My mother's failure had been kept secret to deadly ends.

When the cast is removed my little boy instantly runs down the office hallway. Ecstatic to move freely, he jumps and hops. "No physical therapy needed here!" remarks the orthopedist, delighted with a job well done. No return visit necessary. All that's left of the accident are a few pictures of Ben in his turtle shell—and for me, my memories of the acute feeling of relief when he came out from the general anesthesia that was necessary when they casted his body. Now a teenager, he's strong and agile on the soccer field. No fear, no lasting damage. He flings his body to block shots as goalkeeper, sprints out of reach of opposing players as a mid-fielder. I love to watch him play. It is possible for painful events to be over, to belong to the past, to cause no lasting trauma. Ben's accident did not metastasize into a malignancy that continued to mutate over time.

I did not become my mother. I ended the cycle of abuse not unlike the two mothers who had attacked each other over multiple lifetimes finally ended theirs. Once I disentangled my anger from her violence, I no longer needed it as armor from abuse in a distant past. I could choose understanding and compassion. I unraveled the violence and anger. Now, I would run to my mother and embrace her, as I would have done at any moment after she died, no matter what. Every cycle is impermanent, every trauma can be unwound. I would put myself back into her arms, trusting she will cradle me, just as the Buddha instructed the mother to put her baby in the arms of the demoness and be free of violence.

3. Oriented by Love

There it is again, a strange tingling in my left hand. Is it the same feeling in my foot? No, it feels more like a numbness than a tingling.

These sensations had been going on for some time before I describe them with some anxiety to a friend. She reasons with me that having a newborn child, teaching full-time as a lecturer at Harvard, and being on my own frequently when my husband has to travel for work, are all causing a strain on my body.

But it feels so strange that I go to my doctor, who suggests an MRI as a way to rule out multiple sclerosis, a disease that often first shows symptoms in a person's early thirties, as I was then. I don't even entertain the possibility that the scans would reveal anything. I feel a strain, sure, but I also draw strength from these things: I finished my PhD, I have my first teaching job, I have a strong marriage, and, most importantly, I am a loving mother to our infant son.

No matter how overwhelmed I felt, no matter how many exhausted tears I cried in that first year of mothering, I never felt out of control. My love for our son, Ben, deepened my commitment to breaking my family's cycles of abuse. As an abuse

survivor, I could imagine causing him harm in the most difficult, exhausted moments, but my determination to hold my
body steady is unshaken. I am on a future-oriented path interconnected with others: my new family, friends, my teachers,
and my students. The trauma of my youth is behind me.

In the days leading up to the MRI scan, I optimistically hope
those interconnections will ensure that this path I am on will
unfold into the future of my choosing. My life is oriented toward
keeping Ben safe and creating the conditions for his flourishing.
Ed and I brought him home from the hospital in New York City
on 9/11/2001, that terrifying day of the attack on the Twin Tow-
ers. It made it all too clear to us that many conditions would be
out of our control. But whichever conditions we could shape,
we would.

On the eve of my MRI, I am alone with Ben; Ed is traveling
for work. Charlie and his wife, Janet, anticipated the potential
dangers better than I did, and they invited me to dinner to make
sure I was not alone. I remember thinking that it was a kind but
unnecessary invitation. I was so naive then.

❧

That first MRI scan is strange. I've had so many now, eighteen
years later, that I can even fall asleep during a scan, even though
being in the MRI machine feels like lying in a metal tube that is
being jack-hammered on all sides. Sometimes the sound vibra-
tions are so strong they make my body bounce on the table;
not helpful when I'm desperately determined to keep my body,
and particularly my head, still, in order to get the best images
possible. In the first years the radioactive dye injected into my
arm to show contrast between cancerous and noncancerous

cells makes me nauseous. The possibility of throwing up inside the scan tube with my head inside a plastic steadying cage feels unreasonable—beyond what feels manageable—but I manage.

A neurologist at Mount Auburn Hospital in Cambridge calls the next day to set an appointment to discuss the images. In the office, she shows me and Ed images of my brain. That's pretty wild, we think. We quickly get over enjoying this new x-ray vision as the doctor focuses on a tumor in the posterior of the right frontal lobe of my brain. It's big.

Ed and I fall into a shocked silence. This is when I gasp, "But I have a one-year-old baby!"

It turns out that my long-held fear had been misdirected. While I worried about repeating the cycles of abuse and harming my own child, I hadn't considered the other fearful possibility; like me, Ben would be a motherless child. He would feel what it is to grow up without a mother. Yes, my childhood became less volatile after my mom's death; but it also became emptier and lonelier. I deeply missed the loving and attentive parts of her.

A biopsy follows a few months later. I am awake throughout it so that the surgeons could make sure they weren't cutting into my motor strip. "No! Not there!" I clearly hear the chief neurosurgeon instruct one of the residents.

In order to guide the drill they screw a metal cage-like structure into my scalp. Later, they decide that the most thorough way to be sure they biopsy the right spot in my brain is to do another MRI with the steadying cage still screwed in place.

At other points during the surgery we exchange jokes: "How many neurosurgeons does it take to screw in a light bulb? Just one. They hold the light bulb; the world revolves around them." I counter with "Why did the Buddha make a bad vacuum salesman? Because he had no attachments." Joking during my own brain surgery? It helps ratchet down the stress level.

"We were definitely in the right spot," the chief of neurosurgery announces confidently to my husband and me the next day. "You won the lottery!" the chief resident, proclaims with genuine delight. "We didn't find any malignant cells!"

Where the surgeons give us a "no" to the clear-cut "yes or no" question of whether there was cancer, the oncologist is not convinced. He adds a "maybe" box, which gives rise to many more nuanced questions without simple answers.

The initial scans contained every indicator of a cancerous tumor, but the biopsy found no biological evidence that the tumor was malignant. Because of the tumor's proximity to my motor strip, there was no surgical option at that time, and the other treatment protocols would have caused damage too. The oncologists caution us to just leave it alone. "It is cancer," he definitively proclaims, "but we can't do anything about it."

While waiting for my post-op appointments, I catch a snippet of conversation that sometimes plays back in my memory. A young woman's voice: "My tumor was stable for ten years, *ten years*, and now this!"

Twelve years later, when my tumor awakened, I remember this young woman's voice and words. Had she been a *dakini*, a Tibetan female messenger of wisdom, dressed in jeans and a hoodie sweatshirt, giving me an important vision of my future? Her message that my brain would keep changing stayed with me. It was a warning against complacency and against resisting the reality of this embodied truth of impermanence inside my brain.

In the intervening years I have an MRI scan every two months after that surgery to biopsy my brain tumor, then every six months, then yearly, to keep an eye on what my expert and deeply humane oncologist, Dr. Lai, calls my indolent tumor. Scan after scan, my tumor remains stable. Dr. Lai tells me I am the hopeful case he holds up for his patients the first time he discusses their newly discovered tumors.

In 2014, twelve years after the first MRI, my scan shows that my lazy tumor is now active, busy producing cancerous cells. Malignant. Dr. Lai tells me that my luck has run out for now. There could be a next round of luck in the future.

The surgeon who removes the now-growing tumor sees where that biopsy path twelve years earlier had gone: the needle extracting brain tissue had missed the malignant tumor by a millimeter. They had biopsied healthy brain tissue. That millimeter gave us twelve years of life living with a tumor that looked on scans like a cancerous brain tumor but which wasn't acting like one. During those years, my tumor caused a low level of fear. Most of the time I kept that fear in a mental box up on a shelf in the corner of my everyday reality, with ordinary wonders and meaning. The box had to come down off the shelf each time I had an MRI, but it was easily tucked away again afterward.

Because of that millimeter I had lived all those years without a cancer diagnosis. If the first surgeon had found the tumor and I'd been diagnosed with cancer all those years ago, at a time without a real path of treatment, would I have had the courage to live my life as I had? Would Ed and I have had our second child, Rebekah? Would I have been able to focus on developing my life as a professor and a scholar? Even if my cancer had developed in exactly the same way, would I have been able to live with the fear that a clear diagnosis of brain cancer would have brought, and with the uncertainty of the prognosis?

Those twelve years were a gift. Because of a biopsy's near miss, I carried only the fear of a lazy tumor. Soon after the initial round of tests in 2002, another compassionate oncologist, Dr. Asha Das, in response to my apprehension over the big unknowns in our lives, had encouraged me to have a second child. She explained that some studies showed that pregnancy kept brain tumors from progressing. Further, she told me that even if my tumor became life-taking, my two children would have each other. That last part, that my kids would have each other after I die, is a very loving perspective.

During my last appointment before my daughter is born my obstetrician tells me with her usual certainty that although she would not be on call that weekend I need not worry, since the baby would not be coming in the next few days. I am two days past my delivery date, but she sees no signs of imminent labor.

Yet as I drive home, I feel a sudden overpowering surge of joy. The emotion has a distinct physical sensation, a welling up into my chest and beyond into the crown of my head, transforming into an inner shower of elation and blissful energy—an unfamiliar feeling any time, much less at the very end of a pregnancy. My daughter is on her way. I feel it. I know it.

Labor begins within four hours and lasts another fourteen. The feelings of joy keep fear at bay. My friends Kelly and Simon and their beagle, Willa, walk with me in slow circles around my neighborhood in hopes that it will encourage my labor along.

Ed and I had darkly joked that there would probably be a catastrophic earthquake in the days following her birth; we now lived in southern California, and Ben's birth in New York City, a few days before 9/11, had left us with the fear that disaster would again rapidly follow after joy. But, we admit, the universe does not revolve around us. The normality of the days following Rebekah's birth reassures us that trauma doesn't follow us around like a cartoon-like black cloud.

When my tumor wakes up Rebekah is still a child, hardly ready to process the indeterminacy of our situation. She has a clear and reasonable need for me to stay alive and help her get through high school and prepare for college. While I reassure her the best I can, all I have is this: "I will do anything and everything I can to be alive for you." These are years when a girl needs her mother so intensely. Years when I didn't have my own mom.

One night, while we try to place ourselves on our dying/ living timeline, we cling to each other, faces red from crying and flowing snot, Ben, who is about to graduate high school, comes into Rebekah's room, and he puts a hand on her shoulder. "What's up?" he asks with genuine concern. Rebekah looks at him, managing between sobs to get out, "I don't want Mom to die." "What!? Mom's dying!?" He looks stunned. The kids connect the dots in their own ways; they see what they can take in. I tell them what they ask and want to know.

I repeat to them what Dr. Das had said to me so many years earlier, urging me to live my life fully. I told them, "No matter what happens and when, you have each other . . ." Ben knew this: "Of course, Rebekah. You always have me." Her brother commits himself to a future that's inevitable, maybe coming when they are still too young, maybe when it feels too early no matter how old they are. Our love is here now, and it is a part of their future, whether I am a living part of it or not.

❧

I always try to remind myself that my children are not mine, they are themselves. Our lives are conditions for each other, but while we will never not be connected, we will be one among an infinite variety of conditions that will always be transforming.

How would the impermanence of my body, particularly the tumor in my brain, affect them? It is an ever-present fear; sometimes in my mental box, up on a shelf in my mind, sometimes with me in an MRI scanner, at other times in open conversations with Dr. Lai when I repeat my oft-asked question of "When?" When will this cancer mutate into the condition of my death?

There is no one or right answer, other than we will all continue to change, as will our relationships. The only constant is love, and while love will evolve as we change, I feel certain that it will always be connecting us in some way or another. Amida's golden chain of love tells me this. The Karmapa's presence of universal compassion teaches me this, as do so many other visions into/from the Dharma.

❧

I learn how to sit down next to people I can trust. I closely hold on to the testimony of the nun Uttama, who said, "I approached the nun; she seemed like someone I could trust." Repeating that wise nun's message over and over, my imagination helps me hear more: find people you can trust, sit beside them in friendship, behind them as a student, bow in front of them as a devotee. These trusted friends lead me to others. Remaining open to forming new connections, I have gathered important guides and supports for confronting some of the conditions shaping my life. I find the best oncologist for me, Dr. Lai, and I have confidence in his care. I tell him he is my general contractor of cancer. He advises me on clinical trials, treatment protocol, and when and where I have my craniotomies. I also imagine him as one of the nuns in the *Therigatha*: "I sit in the doctor's exam room, learning what he sees in my brain; he seems like someone I could trust."

My *kalyanamitra*, my spiritual friend, Venerable Damcho Diana Finnegan, is an American nun in the Tibetan tradition. She has steered me to highly auspicious places where we have sat together. Sometimes I sit beside her, other times behind. I first met Damcho when she was studying with Charlie who was then at University of Wisconsin–Madison. I am still at Harvard when Charlie directs her there to use the libraries. He asks me to help her arrange her stay in Cambridge. I, of course, immediately agree. Charlie taught me a professional ethic that has shaped the way I study Buddhist texts and the ways in which I aspire to live my academic relationships: support each other, collaborate, learn from one another.

I find Damcho a place to stay and get her access to the Harvard libraries. She comes to my apartment for meals and holds Ben in her arms, and we become friends. A few years later she stays in my Redlands home and teaches Ben, then a toddler, to protect all life forms, jumping with him over trails of ants. Observing the age-old Buddhist custom of "merit release," we visit a local pet store to buy earthworms, depositing them in my yard and at local parks to save them from a death as bait.

Damcho forms a significant part of Rebekah's life from the beginning. In a favorite photo of the two of them Damcho holds Rebekah in her arms, both look at the camera, both with bald heads. For years, as she wanders the globe teaching Dharma, she visits our home.

In June 2008 Damcho phoned. "You have to come to Seattle." His Holiness the Seventeenth Karmapa, Ogyen Trinley Dorje, was giving teachings and empowerments. The event was a part of his first teaching tour in the United States. I knew of the Karmapa, the head of the Karma Kagyu school, one of the major traditions of Tibetan Buddhism, but at the time I have no personal connection to him. Just twenty-three years old, he is the latest incarnation in a line of exalted teachers stretching back nine hundred years. I am in California, busy with work as a college professor. And as a mother; Ben and Rebekah were still very young. "I don't think I can do it," I tell her. "Too much going on."

"No," she insists. "This is really important; you need to come." In a completely full thousand-seat theater she sits in the front section with other monastics, and I sit behind her in the lay section. Together we receive the Karmapa's teaching and two empowerments.

This begins my connection to the Karmapa. Through my relationship with Damcho, my relationship with His Holiness grows in unimaginable ways over the years.

Three years later, in 2011, at the age of twenty-five years, the Karmapa proposes to have sustained conversations with his generational peers from different countries in order to share their concerns and hopes for their world. At that time the Karmapa is not often traveling away from India, and to make these meetings happen he invites groups of students to his home at Gyuto Monastery, outside of Dharamsala, India. Damcho, who is working with the Karmapa on the program, provides a list of potential university partners in the United States, a list which includes, at my request, the University of Redlands in Southern California, where I teach. Damcho tells me that after hearing the names of the schools and her descriptions he withdrew into a meditative state. Opening his eyes several minutes later he said, "California. It's that one, the one from California." Meaning Redlands. Where I teach. I don't presume to know why he chose my school. Perhaps we had a school calendar that allowed for students to travel to India for a month-long period of time. Maybe he sensed the productive possibilities in my friendship with Damcho. Because of me and her, this opportunity.

In May of 2012 I bring seventeen students to spend almost a month with the Karmapa in his residence in India. My relationship to Buddhism has always had different facets: student, scholar, college teacher. While all of those remained, beginning with this trip to India, I move into a new space of trust deepening into faith. Hour after hour Damcho and I sit side by side on the floor of the Karmapa's personal library surrounded by my students, whose open minds and hearts inspire me each day to bring my full and best self to our conversations.

Throughout my stay, and the one that followed two years later, in 2013, with a second group of students, the subtle fear of my brain tumor remains where I place it, in its mental box. My full being is present in every moment of those conversations with the Karmapa. Listening to his responses to the students' questions, first on foundational Buddhist concepts such as interdependent origination and karma, and then his dynamic teachings on a path to gender justice or sustainable action for creating a compassionate world, I can feel my mind and heart expanding.

In our first two-hour session with the Karmapa, he describes the concept of dependent origination, or *pratityasamutpada*. I lean over to Damcho and whispered in her ear, "I feel like I'm inside a sutra." I am receiving the Dharma directly from an extraordinary person, a man I came to see as a living embodiment of the Dharma, a completely genuine, authentic human being.

Damcho, my students, and I quickly form a heartfelt community of a unique kind, one made possible by the intersection of the expansive compassion of the Karmapa and the open hearts of the students, myself included. From the moment Damcho had told me I had been selected to lead students to meet with the Karmapa, I had wondered why I had been given such an opportunity, questioning whether I deserved such an incredible gift. I came to see the response to these questions in the birth of our new community of open hearts. It wasn't that we had done anything particular to earn it. It wasn't us; we weren't special. Anyone with an open heart and mind and genuine aspirations to put what they learn into service for others is deserving.

Both times I brought students to spend time with the Karmapa he quickly zeroed in on students I know to be privately carrying heavy loads of suffering. One had struggled with drug abuse, another had a painful relationship with their parents, another was questioning their sexual orientation, and another lived with occasionally debilitating depression. I had shared none of this information with anyone, not with Damcho or the Karmapa. Yet somehow he seemed to see them. His attentiveness to these particular individuals was palpable. I noticed it by how he rested his gaze upon them, and how he interwove comments that seemed directed just at them in the flow of our conversation.

These students felt his care too. Some of them confided to me after a particular discussion that they felt he had spoken to them, and them alone, even as we all sat together. He also gave all of us the gift of his own vulnerability; he shared what it felt like for him to live outside of Tibet, having escaped to India at the age of fourteen. In Tibet he had faced increasing political pressure from the Chinese government, and he had needed to study with teachers who could complete his traditional education and training. The Karmapa hadn't seen his parents for over a decade. He spoke several times of his love for them and how much he missed them. He shared that he often felt lonely. His openness showed us that even the most extraordinary people carry difficult experiences and emotions. It is a teaching on courage for me. I draw upon it often when I share my cancer experiences with others and while I write this book.

That close connection we developed was in part the result of bringing the right conditions with us to India. Some of those conditions were formal and ritualistic. In order to convey respect and gratitude for this opportunity, the students consented to act according to norms that would signal respect to the Tibetans working for and around the Karmapa. These included dressing modestly and relatively formally; standing when the Karmapa entered the room; sitting lower than him; keeping voices low in the monastery; being intentional about how much space our group was occupying in those places. These were not superficial actions, and our hosts clearly appreciated the efforts taken by young U.S. students to attend to Tibetan cultural norms of respect.

Each student's preparations also included giving a personal gift to the Karmapa, delivered at our first meeting. Following the Tibetan practice of bringing an offering to a teacher, I asked my students to bring a gift that shared a bit of who they were as well as that expressed their understanding of who the Karmapa was. On our second interview some of their gifts were displayed on the shelves around his library. His staff of Tibetan monks took time to look at them, seeming to acknowledge the heart-to-heart connections.

Maybe this helped to make sense of the Karmapa's break from some aspects of protocol later into our stay. On a few occasions he sat on the floor with the students or played instruments—including one made for him by one of the students. They shared a lot of laughter with him, and in fact his attendant privately told me it had been a long time since he had heard the Karmapa laugh so much.

As the Karmapa admitted to us, Tibetans don't really conceive of him as an ordinary person. This is understandable in a Tibetan context: he was identified at the age of seven as the seventeenth reincarnation of the first Karmapa, who had lived nine hundred years before. From that perspective he was nine hundred years old, a figure of immense authority and reverence. From another perspective, he was twenty-five years old, just a few years older than these students who travel to spend time with him. They shared common interests such as a fondness for comic books (especially Marvel), music, and painting. Yet unlike our students, who had the freedom to decide who they are, what they would do, and how they wanted to live, the Karmapa's life was set out for him at the young age when he was recognized. While the students worked hard to understand this, perhaps they brought a gift of freedom to the Karmapa, who maybe caught a glimpse of himself through their eyes as a person who really was just twenty-five years old.

In 2013 I brought a second group of students to Gyuto for another series of conversations with His Holiness. During those weeks he taught us the benefits and challenges of community through stories from *The Life of Milarepa*. This text is integral to one of his communities; it is his and other Tibetan lamas' responsibilities to care for and preserve Milarepa's teaching for the living communities of today. That responsibility, he taught us, is to cultivate virtue and the awareness of interconnection.

These are perspectives I now desperately need as I struggle to accept the care I require as my illness progresses.

It was quite an experience to hear the Karmapa's retelling of Milarepa's life story, as he sat in front of a large, extremely beautiful painting of Milarepa. When his lesson on community finished, we waited for the Karmapa to rise, and then we stood, bowed, and quietly followed him out of the library. As our group prepared to leave from the building's lobby, a huge bird flew into sight and settled down on a low concrete wall just outside the building. One student identified it as a species of vulture. Another reminded us of the story of how Milarepa's master, Marpa, had received a vision that had predicted the future of his lineage: four pillars each served as the resting place for a particular animal; Milarepa's pillar was topped with a vulture.

What did it mean? I suggested that signs of the Buddha, Dharma, and Sangha—the three jewels of Buddhism, its three refuges—are living resources all around us. They not only are a part of the storied past, but are actively inviting us in. Each of us would choose what to make of these experiences. I did encourage them to remember the Karmapa's storytelling and this vulture. Perhaps if they saw a vulture at another time and place, say, in the American Southwest, they might invite their imaginations to move between their present moment, the far distant mythical past when Marpa gave this vision to Milarepa, and this moment in India when we shared time and space with His Holiness in India.

One day, during the first visit in 2011, the students and I joined the Karmapa for a short excursion outside of the monastery—a visit to nearby Norbulingka, a Tibetan cultural arts center with a beautiful temple on its grounds. It was a clear blue-sky day. After some time inside the temple he suggested we gather closely on the temple's steps for a group photo. Word had gotten out that the Karmapa was at Norbulingka. Since it wasn't common for him to be seen outside of Gyuto Monastery, hundreds of Tibetans had quickly appeared, eager to see him—and to be seen by him.

As we stood on the steps to take the group photo, the crowd, acting the role of a spiritual paparazzi, photographed him too. While all of this was going on, a perfect white and fluffy cloud appeared out of nowhere in that still perfectly blue sky and drifted right above us. For a moment or two it dropped warm, large raindrops only on our heads. No rain fell outside of that little space we occupied.

It was a funny moment that quickly came and went. Perhaps a few people look up, but I guess most don't notice anything. I can still see the whole tiny scene unfold. It feels to me as if I'd been drawn into a set piece from any number of stories. In literature such a phenomenon can be called "a rain of flowers." It is a response of the earth to a moment of goodness and compassion.

Feeling the warmth of the water on my arms, I look at

Damcho; we both looked at the Karmapa. He smiles at us and points at the sky. With a little mischievousness, he says, "Now look for the rainbow."

⚮

What if we could cultivate our imaginations to serve as bridges into any Buddhist narrative? What story might you choose? It would be impossible for me to limit myself, but one would be the story of the dying mother of the Buddha, Maya, as told in popular Khmer folk traditions. I see Prajapati, Maya's sister, holding her hand, stroking her cheek, maybe placing her newborn son on his mother's chest. I imagine her softly saying to her older, dying sister, "He will be fully loved, well cared for, you will always be with him, I will always be here for you."

A year after my second trip to India I face my first major brain surgery. Damcho is able to let the Karmapa know about the growth of my tumor and my upcoming surgery, and she asked him for practice advice. He told her which mantras we should recite.

Devotion allows us to carry the object of that devotion wherever we go. Just two weeks after receiving his advice, Ed and I sit in the pre-op waiting room, jam-packed with people anxiously waiting to be called up for their surgery. It feels more like a crowded train platform, the worst kind of setting for me, since I get anxious and distracted in crowds. I close my eyes and silently recite my mantras using prayer beads blessed by the Karmapa during one of my trips to India. Suddenly I deeply feel his presence enter that crowded room. Opening my eyes a tiny bit, I see him in the doorway. After the image fades, I whisper to my husband, "Is His Holiness here? I thought I saw him."

"No." He gently answers without judgment. Of course he wasn't there, but I feel his presence. My moment of reverie shifts but doesn't leave me. I feel surrounded by it going into surgery and recovering afterward.

In post-op, I remained unconscious from the general anesthesia for longer than usual. The intensive care nurses had a hard time bringing me back from total unconsciousness. Nevertheless, or perhaps fearing the worst, the nurse brought my husband and father in to see me as soon as possible.

It proved to be too soon; they had waited anxiously through the six-hour procedure but waiting longer would have been much easier than seeing me in that unconscious state. Ed later told me that my eyes were open but that I seemed totally gone. It frightened my father so much that he left; he just couldn't see me that way. It looked like I was dead.

In March 2015, His Holiness embarked on a tour of university campuses in the United States, for which invitations from universities piled up. The Karmapa was told he could not fit all of them into his trip, and he allowed his team to decline whichever invitations they could not accommodate. He said the University of Redlands, however, had to stay on his itinerary.

My colleagues and our administrators at the university gave their full support, and really their hearts, to welcome him to our campus with the appropriate honor. The facilities crew strung hundreds of strands of Tibetan prayer flags around the university grounds, most spectacularly between the tops of the pillars in front of the chapel. Campus security suggested flying the Karmapa's "dream flag" below the American flag. The university bestowed on him the honorary degree of Doctorate of Humane Letters in the packed chapel, filled to capacity with many Buddhist sanghas and Tibetans living in California.

When our eyes first met at my home upon his arrival to Redlands, his first words are "Your health?" His typically brief question invites me to provide as much detail as I wish to describe. A moment later when we are sitting in the very ordinary space of my kitchen. I say, "I am OK," although my mouth is full of sores from the experimental chemotherapy I am taking.

His reply to my "OK" cuts right through my artifice: "It was like you were dead but then you were no longer dead." I immediately know that he is referring to my lengthy post-operative unconsciousness. How did he know? Damcho doesn't know; she hasn't told him. Had other things happened to my consciousness during the surgery or after that I don't know about? I didn't ask, and he did not elaborate. By communicating that he knew of my unconscious state during and after the surgery, it seems to me, he was letting me know that he was present, just as I had felt him to be. I may lack the ability to be in his physical presence all the time, but I feel that no matter the distance, he is present for me, and in many different ways. My work is to both deepen and broaden my mind to be aware of those precious gifts of care and commitment. And to receive that presence with humility and gratitude.

Is all this my own imagination, arrogance, and clinging to illusions? That may very well be the case. None of my stories about the Karmapa reveals anything about me. What I hope to express is the presence of living compassion in our world, in our time, by the Karmapa, and of course, by many other Buddhist masters. Stories of such virtuous beneficence don't only belong in the past; they originate in our present too. Reading the stories from the Buddhist canon or later Buddhist literary traditions helps me be prepared for them in my own experience now. In a way, Karmapa is teaching me to read my own life narrative, not only from my own self-reflections but from reflections outside of myself.

In the midst of that busy visit to Redlands in 2015 the Karmapa makes time for short private audiences before the degree cere-mony at which he delivers a public address to 1,500 people. I too have a short private, formal audience.

His gaze of complete presence falls on me, and he makes his usual invitation for me to speak: "Yes?" His Holiness asks. "My only concern is for my children," I say. "I know what it is to grow up without a mother, and I worry for them." Medita-tive silence followed. Opening his eyes from what appears to me to be a movement of his consciousness through time, he holds me in his gaze and says, in what I was coming to realize was his pattern of direct communication, "They will be fine. OK?" "OK," I repeat (or plead). And that was all. The next day as my family and I have a brief private goodbye at our home, His Holiness holds out his arms to my son and daugh-ter, beckoning them to approach. "Come closer," he gently instructs them. Towering over them, he holds them close to him, encircling them with his arms. I stand before them. He again looks directly into my eyes, holding me in his gaze. Now I understood his response to me the day before. They will be fine, no matter when I die. There are many conditions of love. I was one, but just one, of those conditions. I feel his assurance that they will have the conditions to flourish. Maybe he will be one of those conditions, maybe he knows that others will be present and available to them. This moment gives me a vitally important condition I need to live fully with my cancer, no matter the speed of the cancer, no matter the length of my future.

And indeed, the pace of impermanence picked up again. Two years later my tumor changed again, as they always do; brain tumors are a particularly rich embodiment of impermanence. The tumor grew and revealed itself to be a much more aggressive form of cancer than we had previously hoped.

Before the treatment of the progressing disease began, I made a quick, five-day trip to India for the formal launch of His Holiness the Karmapa's book *Interconnected: Embracing Life in Our Global Society*, which Damcho and I had edited. The book had grown out of the conversations between His Holiness and my students. For the year and a half that we worked on the book, his teachings lived in my heart and at the forefront of my mind. His confidence that we could reshape the teachings he gave during our conversations into the fluidity of a monograph written for every reader bolstered my confidence in myself. I grew confident that from the depth of my connection to my lama grew an ability to be of service through him to people who, like me, welcome his teachings into their daily lives.

I had just completed participation in a two-year trial for a new chemotherapy drug. The very last scan showed ambiguous images of new tumor growth. It hadn't worked. In a quickly found moment that offered a private audience, I told the Karmapa of the likelihood of another craniotomy and then radiation and chemotherapy treatments. After telling him what would soon be happening to me, I verbalized my aspiration for how I hoped to live through it: "I want to be oriented by love rather than fear." "Yes," he said, nodding as he looked me in the eyes. In that moment I set my orientation toward a path for living a meaningful life with compassion, and my lama, the Karmapa, confirmed it. I know my way forward. His affirmation deepened my courage to believe in it. It deepened my faith in my capacity to make it the guiding principle of my life in my last few years, and now, the central theme of this book.

I am a person of ill-fortune, and a person of great good fortune.

4. Living with Uncertainty: When Will I Die?

Aseries of oncologists, beginning with that first arrogant oncologist I saw in Boston in 2002, told me there was something in my brain that looked just like a cancerous tumor but wasn't acting like one. Because biopsies of the brain are such invasive procedures, there wasn't a compelling reason for doing another. Even if they had found cancerous cells there wasn't much they could have done at the time. The tumor was so close to my motor strip that surgery or radiation posed too great a risk, and, given my young age, it wasn't worth taking the chance.

The only thing to do, I was told, was to monitor the tumor regularly to see if it was changing; malignant tumors usually do so at a rapid pace. So that's what we did. For more than a decade I lived with the awareness that I had a brain tumor of some sort, but I didn't know whether or not it would eventually cause me harm. Living with this great unknown was hard, as I told Dr. Lai at every checkup; but as he correctly said, certainty could only be bad news. When certainty finally presented itself after my craniotomy in 2014, which resulted in a diagnosis of grade II brain cancer, the clarity of diagnosis did not bring the paradoxical relief I had anticipated. I would have preferred the uncertainty. Surgery that year removed 90 percent of the tumor. The 10 percent remaining lay so closely to my motor strip that the surgeon felt she had no choice but to leave it in place. Again, there would be no clear prognosis. A grade II diagnosis signified that the cancer cells were mutating, but not as rapidly as they could be on the scale that reaches grade IV. That would come later.

The doctors at the UCLA tumor board did not reach consensus on the next steps of my treatment. The surgeon recommended moving ahead with radiation and chemotherapy, as was the standard protocol. But others on the treatment team argued that since the diagnosis was of low-grade cancer, I had time before I had to decide whether or not to go through the brutal treatment with its potentially debilitating side effects. Yet again the advice I got was that I should just wait and do nothing. My cancer was now malignant; doing nothing was nearly unbearable for me. The vagaries of my place in time, the impermanence in my body, left me emotionally adrift. I didn't know how to temporally frame my life. The averages of human life span no longer seem to apply to me, given the fatality rates of this cancer. At forty-four was I approaching middle-age, or was I in the final stage of my life?

Although I decided against radiation and chemo, because of the severity of their side effects vs. proven results, trying something, anything, would make it possible for me to direct myself toward a future. I therefore signed up to participate in a clinical trial for an experimental chemotherapy drug at the University of California, San Francisco. I committed to a one-year trial but ended up staying on it for two, from early 2015 to early 2017. Over the course of the trial the remnants of the tumor remained stable, and the chemo caused some seriously annoying side effects that I was able to manage. I felt like I was living responsibly with my cancer.

During the trial I had to do MRI scans every two months. I often saw the same fellow patients at the MRI center and in the waiting room at the oncologists. Some were much older than me , others considerably younger. Waiting for the results of the latest view into my brain slowed time into prolonged periods of silence when all I could do is stare at the beautiful view of the San Francisco Bay and the Golden Gate Bridge, holding Ed's hand and silently saying my mantra.

This was my two-month cycle, which built up at home with escalating uneasiness before the trip from Southern California and culminated with the MRI test and the wait for the oncologist to give us either the bad news, that the tumor was active, or what counted as good news, that the tumor was stable, for now.

During one of these visits, a couple—younger, fitter, more beautiful than us—were called back to the exam room before we went in. After a long time, the woman (I assume the wife of the patient) hurried through the waiting room to the restroom looking down to shield her grief-strained, horrified face. Would that be Ed in a few moments? Would my scans show a rapidity of growth, the next slice in our amputated future? Why that woman's husband instead of me? Or did the knowing-not-knowing always lead to this moment in time, at some time or other? Living with a terminal cancer meant the only knowable answer is: I struggle living daily with the question *when*?

"Why me?" is a stupid question, or more gently, an unproductive one. There are known contributing factors for some forms of cancer, but even then, a causal relationship can't be definitively proven. And anyway, it can seem like blaming the victim. We get sick and we die because of impermanence. There is no arguing with that foundational Buddhist teaching.

"When?" is a question most people avoid. Or answer by assuring themselves and others that their time is a long way off. As though not knowing the time of death guarantees that it is nowhere near to now. This question comes into sharper focus when the conditions leading to death are known, felt, and directly shaping one's daily patterns of living.

I've largely (but not completely) avoided the "why," but figuring out how to live with the "when" is very hard. Those series of two months between brain scans initially brought some relief—even comfort—in their regularity, and in the fact that we would leave San Francisco with the news that the tumor was still stable. But then, a few days before the checkup process approached, my horizon would begin to feel unstable again. There is forward motion, but it felt like I was constantly stumbling, tripping as I moved toward the next MRI looking for changes in the tumor as the sign or progression of the cancer.

My honest, ethical doctors are upfront about the imprecision of the available tools for making these assessments. Ed refers to the MRI measurement tools as Etch a Sketches, as they appear on the computer screen like our childhood toys. In any case, my repeated pleas for a prognosis are dependent on the interpretation of when all this began. Time, again, is the issue. "When" isn't just a matter of conclusion, but of the start of all this as well. When did they arise, these conditions that created the present and are determining my future? When did my brain cancer begin? Was I born with it? Unlikely. Did it begin when my mom broke the bottle on my skull? Impossible to know. When I am injured in the car accident that killed my mom? Some doctors consider that possibility, others give a definitive no. Most of us live with uncertainty of how to frame the time of our lives and life experiences.

The way we live in time is a condition for living well. My visceral memories of my past made possible the work of setting down my anger and fear. While I no longer cling to those memories, or at least to the pain of those events, they continue to help me know the conditions of my present and shape my concerns for the future too. I often hear or read that people who experience severe illness, or an event that brought death into focus, gain a new appreciation for living in the present moment. That's great, but I'm not sure I totally buy it. Or it doesn't release me from a more complicated relationship to the time frame of my life.

When does our "when" begin? In many worldviews—religious or philosophical—it is at birth. But what about before that? The Buddhist process of rebirth is an opaque filter, another form of knowing that there is much we do not know about ourselves. We know that we generated karma in pasts that far preceded our birth into this life, but we do not, and cannot, know anything about the causes of that karma or its current effects. Only the buddhas know such a thing; the Pali texts tell us that the vision to see our own and others' past and future lifetimes is gained only on the second stage of awakening.

So, again, is the question of when this illness began a productive question? From a doctor's perspective it is relevant for both diagnosis and prognosis. This is one of the interpretive levers that makes my future unfixable: Do we take as the cancer's starting point that MRI in 2002 that first shows the tumor? Or the 2014 craniotomy that brings me the diagnosis of grade II glioma brain cancer? Or does the clock reset in 2017, with the second craniotomy that diagnoses grade IV glioblastoma, one of the deadliest forms of cancer? If doctors start the measurement of my prognosis in 2014 or earlier, then my current longevity goes beyond any of the statistical charts. If 2017, then my prognosis probabilities are scarier; I may be dead when you are reading this. My oncologists don't know with absolute certainty when the beginning begins.

I find myself shifting between these different temporal contexts quite often in my attempts to accept the uncertainty as a primary dimension of impermanence. My pole star is my children. How old will they be in two years? In six? In ten? I've told my oncologist that my goal is to live until my youngest leaves home for college. His nod acknowledges that hope, but he can't responsibly reassure me that this cancer, at least, won't be the obstacle to reaching that goal. He cannot predict the success of my aspiration.

My progressively dire diagnoses and my decreasingly hopeful prognoses have created a new and distressing relationship with time. I long to live within the structures of Buddhist stories when a buddha predicts the future, in particular, those stories, found in many Theravada and Mahayana scriptures, that offer a bodhisattva—a buddha-to-be—a detailed blueprint of their future.

The most famous story in Theravada literature of a bodhisattva's prediction of future buddhahood is made by the buddha Dipamkara to our Buddha, Siddhartha Gautama. Once upon an unimaginably long time ago, the bodhisattva who would become Shakyamuni Buddha was a young man named Sumedha, who in adulthood renounced his life as a householder after the death of his wealthy parents. Seeing the meaninglessness of wealth in the face of their death, he gives it all away and retreats to a solitary, ascetic life in the mountains.

One day, news reaches him that a buddha, Dipamkara, was on his way to the village far below him. Dressed only in a bark cloth, Sumedha descends by means of his power of flight (attained through his advancement) and joins the crowds preparing the roadways for the arrival of the buddha and his monastic community, or Sangha. Their aim is to make the road perfectly smooth and beautiful as an act of veneration.

Sumedha finds a spot of the road still muddy and unprepared for Dipamkara, who is quickly approaching, and lies down in that mud, making his matted hair and body into a bridge for the buddha and his seemingly infinite line of monks to walk across. Coming to Sumedha's prone form, now prostrate in a posture of worship, the buddha Dipamkara halts his procession, his feet directly pointing at Sumedha's head. In this most auspicious moment of opportunity, Sumedha makes an aspiration for his future: he vows that, in a lifetime so many years away in the future they couldn't be counted, he too would become a buddha, just like the buddha Dipamkara, who then stood upon his hair.

All buddhas are said to embark on the bodhisattva path in this manner: with a vow, made before a buddha, to attain complete and perfect enlightenment for the benefit of all. Upon receiving Sumedha's aspiration, the buddha Dipamkara then fulfilled his role in the story by confirming the vow and providing a prediction of its fulfillment. He closes his eyes and sends his consciousness into an examination of the future. Returning to the present moment, he reports on what he has just seen: in a specific future Sumedha would become the Buddha Shakyamuni. The prediction includes a great many details of the future life when he would live as that buddha, including the names of his family members and the circumstances of his birth, renunciation, and awakening to buddhahood.

Dipamkara's abilities to know the future are accepted by all as a fact of a buddha's omniscience. So much so that everyone who hears it that day shares in the reassurance that this was not just a possible future, but a future that they could be sure of. Moreover, it was a future they could be a part of; those members of the Sangha who lacked the confidence that they could attain liberation in that life vowed that they would do so during the lifetime of Shakyamuni. Dipamkara's prediction gave them certainty of their future too.

I have long been fascinated by the Sumedha story, years before cancer became a condition of my life. I lived with it intimately for months as I wrote about it as the central narrative for my doctoral dissertation. I came to know it in a halting, disrupted way as I attempted to find the best forms of expression in English and translate it from the canonical Pali *Buddhavamsa* and also from medieval Pali commentary. As was appropriate for the task of writing an academic thesis, I was focused on my analytical interpretations of the story for my arguments on relational ethics in Theravada literature. I focused particularly on the relationships of buddhas and bodhisattvas still on the path to awakening. That goal cannot be achieved by an individual alone, I argued, but only through the supporting relationships of many others. In spite of my practiced academic critical distance, the story did become a part of me. I thought of it constantly as I walked around Manhattan, where I then lived. Phrases and words echoed in the background of my mind. Scenes played out for me, on a block ahead of me, on the busy streets of the city, floating above the crowds of people at an intersection waiting on a sidewalk above a muddy gutter.

My own past self, that young, healthy student, attempted to understand the relationships among buddhas. My focus was entirely upon those past, present, and future buddhas. I wasn't much interested in what was happening to all the ordinary people in the crowd around them. Experiencing this story now, my illness brings me into the crowd, a crowd of people who, like me, know that their present is limited and perilously uncertain.

Re-reading this story with my now-shaky grasp of time, I view it from a different perspective. I no longer read it from above with a spotlight on the bodhisattva's aspiration for the future and the buddha's prediction that time will absolutely unfold precisely as foretold. A clear prediction of my remaining time, I had thought, would make my diagnosis and prognosis bearable. As I moved through the stages of treatment, I began to rethink the purpose of the prediction stories that I studied for so long. They were not only for the sake of the bodhisattvas who receive them. They were intended also for those following behind the exalted beings on the path, those people in the crowd who would be reassured by a known future, one in which a buddha would be present to care for them.

This story gives me two possible ways of relating to time: a clear view into a known future and a conditional view that can't tell me anything in absolute terms. I want an unconditional declaration of my future with cancer. In my illness I want my own prediction. I want to know where I stand now in the time frame of my own life. I want the clarity of a definitive prognosis, not the foggy, groggy prognostication of statistical tables. I don't want to pine for the possibility of a new clinical trial opening up in time that might extend my life, should I meet the necessary conditions for that trial. The future that I live toward is infinitesimal compared to the temporal frame of this Buddhist story. I'm not hoping for a geological leap across millions of years in time. I desire to know: will I live for six months or seventeen? For a year or for years? How many? I want to know for certain what this cancer was going to take away from me and when. I want what I cannot know. There is something important in my not-knowing. The impermanence and interconnectedness of time is real. Really real. My cancer makes me see it, deal with it, live with it, grow and transform with it.

❦

The present moment totally encases me when I go through my most intense treatments. Full brain radiation is a sharp arrow pointed at my skull that literally pinned me to each moment as it happens. Waiting for my first radiation appointment after my craniotomy in 2017, I am scared. I act stoically. If I remember correctly, I calmly tell Ed and my best friend, Kelly, that I am fine, that there is no need for anyone to come to the hospital with me. But I am scared. It all seems so freaky. Radiating my brain?!

While I wait for the whole process to begin, I watch a boy, maybe five or six years old, playing at a block toy with lots of moving pieces. His dad, a big man, sits on the floor looking at his son with deep love and presence. Both of them are calm and focused on the toy. There is no terror that could match that of one's child, the heart outside a parent's heart, waiting for radiation treatment to treat the cancer in his young body; no terror that I can imagine greater than this. I pray, "Let me take on whatever illness, whatever suffering this father and son are experiencing. Give it to me."

At an earlier appointment I have a mesh mask made of my head. I am suddenly staring in a horror movie. Straws are placed in my nose for breathing as papier-mâché-like strips of gauze are draped over my face to make the mask. Snaps are then placed on the side of the mask. At the beginning of my first radiation session, and for the seven and a half weeks of radiation treatments that follow, I lay down on a moveable metal table and, in order to line up the scope for the radiation beam, this mask is placed over my face. It is then snapped onto the table and the machine moves over me to beam the radiation directly at my brain.

The technicians who gently and kindly do all this maneuvering instruct me to stay absolutely still, so the radiation would hit the right spot. Still, always I'm told to stay still. Then I am alone with my mask and the radiation.

Breathing and mantra recitation quiets my mind through all of this. There is something about the precision of my body's placement that proves to be perfect for mindfulness practice. I follow my breath from the crown of my head, as it moves through my brain, down through my throat, into my limbs, and downward into my toes. I follow my breath and stay still. Once the radiation beam begins, my internal mantra recitation starts up more or less on its own. It becomes a dynamic practice over those seven-and-a-half weeks. My practice takes on its own form of reverie. Sometimes the Karmapa's cooling moon-like light shields me from the searing beams that leave me burning into the night, bags of frozen peas cooling my scalp. Sometimes I mentally call out to him: "Karmapa Khyenno"—"Karmapa, think of me."

At other times, my mind calls out to Amitabha Buddha, repeating Amitabha's mantra as instructed by the Karmapa—I relish the mirthful nature of my practice. It responds to the present moment as needed. After two or three sessions, I ask the technicians if the lights normally change over the course of a radiation session. "No. It is this same gray light the whole time," they respond.

"What do you see?" they ask with curiosity—other patients have reported seeing different things during radiation, but they have no explanation. I tell them that I see different colors, changing like a light show. First there is a strong white light, then a short period of red light, and finally a steady blue light. I tell my friend Damcho about it, and she explains that it's the same order of lights in Amitabha practice: the practitioner visualizes Buddha Amitabha in the sky in front with those three colored lights flowing out of the buddha's body into her own.

If I were a better practitioner, I would have made the connection myself. Damcho advises me how to connect the radiation lights to the Amitabha practice, and from that point onward I follow her practice instructions: I direct the white light to enter the crown of my head, the red light to enter my throat, and the blue light to enter my heart.

❧

My closest family relationships, like most intimate relationships, are complicated. Faced with my mortality, I begin to see all the ways I had participated in the cause of the hardness, the dysfunction growing from my traumatic childhood family. I decide I had to own my part, and in doing so I furrow new tracks and see that my loved ones are willing to walk a new path with me. I take stock of the time that I need, the time that I want, and the time that I've wasted. My father and sister generously offer to care for me during my cancer treatment; they are willing to be present when I am most vulnerable, when I can't be my defensive self, and that has to be OK. They are sources of care, not harm.

The time that I need: to finish this book and other academic projects can't compare to the time I need to help my children become adults. This is what scares me the most. When I dream of the future I want, it isn't just my time; it's my children's futures too. I dream of helping them raise their young children as they build their own careers, but of course, who knows how they will shape their futures, how they will spin their dreams of love, babies, and careers. I want them to have what I did not—help. Ed and I lived away from our families while we built careers and managed our own family unit. We made it work, even if we felt the absence. We envied the families we knew who dropped kids off with grandparents so they could have a weekend to themselves for whatever reason—to keep some fun in life or just to maintain sanity. We didn't have that, yet we are still married, and our teenage kids are self-directed, kind people. Maybe they already have what they need from me. After I'm gone their father and others will be rich resources. It doesn't have to be me. It's a future I want, but not one I need.

Embodying the impermanence of time alters my mothering for the better too. I've not clung to stages of my kid's lives, measuring each change as they evolve further from childhood and move further away from me. While I work to stay out of the way of their relationship to time as it feels to them, internally I'm trying to catch sight of their future in the present. I do fear that I won't be present at important future moments. Ironically, I grasp at these moments that are not yet here. I purposefully blur my focus at the excitement and frippery of a junior high school prom; can this give me a peek through a time-traveling window of a potential wedding day? Can a ceremony of moving between middle school to high school serve as a small potential substitution for applauding at college graduations I'm unlikely to attend? They are all illusions that placate my measurements of my uncertain future. Keep those illusions in check, I remind myself, and keep them to yourself. I don't want my family, especially my kids, racing into their own futures at a falling pace for my sake.

There are real limits to my ability to be present in my children's lives. Some of these may seem like small things, but they might be significant to them; I'm never the parent who volunteers to drive on crazy Southern California highways to take this or that athletic team to their away games. But I make it to their home games. I nap to offset the heavy fatigue that medication buries me under so that I'll have some energy in the afternoons when they get home. I wear hats and scarves to hide my hair as it falls out in strange patterns from radiation.

My daughter sometimes asks questions about when I'll die as she measures her own time against mine. I honestly don't know the best way to answer. I want to stay within the truth, but I also don't want to scare her unnecessarily, given the tenuousness of what we know and all that we still don't know.

While crying, Rebekah courageously tells me, "I need you to be here until I leave for college. I really need you to be here until then." "Yes. I know. I will do everything I can to be here." I reassure her time after time. I think it is realistic to hope for that. Her courage to face her uncertain future with clarity of what she needs and knowing that she may not get it astounds me. She schedules her own phone meeting with my oncologist, Dr. Lai, to directly ask him her own questions. He generously agrees, and the two of them have their own conversation. Once again my confidence grows deeper that she will be fine, better than fine, in her own future.

My practice during the course of overlapping radiation and chemotherapy has moments of reverie, but the whole thing is still scary and painful. I dread each time I descend through the hospital floors to the sub-basement, the nuclear medicine area. Even so, I reverted to old patterns of refusing help: "I'm fine," I repeat to everyone.

My best friend, Kelly, did go with me one day, as I was moving further into the seven-week treatment regime and the fatigue had thickened. When we got off the elevator, she looked at me closely. "Your whole body just sank; you aren't fine." It is important for me to acknowledge that. I did shuffle through the hallways to the radiation area. And I also gave a happy hello to the technologists I knew by name. They greet me like a friend, complimenting my outfit, asking me what I had planned for the weekend. They generously tried their best to normalize this Frankenstein-like process as much as possible. I attempted to reciprocate their care by being as easy a patient as I could possibly be. I lay perfectly still, always, no whining, no resistance to the pressure of my face mask.

The times my family spends traveling together are my strongest anchors in time. We do without a lot of material things in order to be able to travel the world as a family. We've made adventuring together as a foursome a defining aspect of our eighteen years of life together. We've chosen where we travel in a variety of ways. A December trip to Salzburg where Steve and Kim, our close friends, were living introduced our California kids to real cold and to Christmas markets, where cannon blasts off an old fort mark Christmas Eve. An earlier trip to Australia came from nothing more than a breathless instant of Ed running upstairs: he'd just seen round-trip flights to Sydney for only $450. "Buy them," I said. "We'll figure the trip out later!"

I'm grateful for those moments that arose from jumping into an unexpected opportunity: hot sun on the boat ride back from snorkeling on the Great Barrier Reef when a humpback whale gifted us a show of impossible grace, breaching far out of the water. As if that wasn't enough, the whale circled the catamaran, surfacing to breathe right where I was watching the water, Rebekah in my arms. We look down, the whale looks up. We held each other's eyes for several seconds. Magical! Seeing and being seen! This is an experience I draw upon as I read Buddhist stories describing the wonders and love alive alongside us in the world. We need to train our senses to see, hear, feel them.

Rebekah chose Greece after she'd been reading a book series based on Greek mythology. Disappointment and a little bit of outrage ensued when she saw that fires are no longer lit at the ruins of their ancient temples; the gods and goddesses had been abandoned! Still, kayaking to empty beaches through aquamarine waters softened the blow. Ben and Ed wandered enchanted through the cobblestone streets of the Byzantine city of Mystras. When Ben asked why kings would build so many churches in such a small city, I explained how political leaders displayed religious devotion in order to justify their right to rule. We explore, we teach, we learn, we enjoy. Everywhere we've gone we've experienced kindness; everywhere there is both beauty and suffering.

Friends and family sometimes question why we take the kids with us on our travels. This was especially true when they were very young—three or four years old. It puzzled many why we'd take them on these trips that they wouldn't remember. But we know that the experiences shape their persons, and anyway, *I* remember, and I return to these experiences over and over again to relive precious times of our being in the world together. I hope that the trips that they do remember will be spaces that will help them recall me. I repeat my favorite stories with them hoping to make them robust and long-lived. (Ed's stock answer is simpler: "Well, we love to travel, and they go where we go.")

Two years after my second craniotomy and the conclusion of the experimental chemotherapy, my family traveled to Japan. I had wanted to go there for decades, and it didn't take much to convince the other three. While they loved the energy, imagination, and fun of Tokyo, for me Kyoto was love at first sight. Eikando Zenrinji, an ancient Jodo Shinshu temple, felt like home, and I wanted to remain there for as long as possible. An aspiration for the future formed as we walked through the entry: if I live long enough, I vowed to spend three seasons of a year in Kyoto and pray at the temple every day.

Charlie has given us instructions to see a unique statue of Amitabha—known in Japan as Amida—in this temple. We pass through different shrine rooms and spaces, moving farther up the hill upon which Eikando Zenrinji is built. I hold my breath a little until we got to that upper clearing, nestled in the hillside trees and looking out across the valley. On our way there we duck into a lower, smaller shrine area. While Ed and I are still in the outer entry rooms, our kids came from a rear shrine. Pulling us along with wide eyes, they explain that they found a painting that looked just like the Karmapa. They are spot on. The painting of Yamagoe Amida, the buddha, looks to all of us like a portrait His Holiness the Seventeenth Karmapa. Here he is with us seated before a rising moon, shining cool, gentle light over the hills behind this magnificent Jodo Shinshu temple. Here he is painted as a form of Amida Buddha, bringing gentle light to the world. Anywhere, everywhere there is universal compassion following me, following every one of us. In Tibetan Buddhism the Karmapas are believed to be embodiments of Amitabha.

When we reached the upper altar, nestled in the treetops, I found the statue Charlie sent me to look for and knelt to recite the Amitabha practice given to me by the Karmapa. It is a beautiful small statue of a walking Amida. As he seems to be gliding away from his devotee, he looks back over his shoulder. According to the temple's story, in a version told by the Jodo Shinshu priest Reverend Toshiyuki Umitani, one day the monk Eikan was practicing the *nembutsu* around the shrine of Amida Buddha. This is the practice of chanting "Namo Amida Butsu"—"Homage to the Buddha Amitabha (or Amida)"—as a way to invoke his grace. After Eikan performed this practice for some time, he saw the statue of Amida step down from the shrine and begin to walk right in front of him. He was so surprised that he halted the ritual on the spot, staring in awe. Amida turned and looked back over his left shoulder, calling to him in a soft voice, "Eikan, ososhi"—"Eikan! Follow me!" or "Eikan! You're so slow!"

Imagine the encouragement and comfort. No matter how slowly I move in my debilitated state, Amitabha urges me on. I'm right in front of you, Amitabha tells me; if you reach out your hand, you'll find mine.

Seeing this image and learning its story led me to a different experience of my unknown future. Freeing myself of my desire to know a future I can't know, I could surrender myself with the promise of being caught in the waiting arms of Amitabha and taken to Sukhavati, his Land of Bliss. I just have to let go.

As my faith grows, so will my courage and trust. Moments that seem disconnected—direct times shared with the Karmapa, reverie in radiation sessions, coming to understand the presence of compassionate care from my mother through what I learn in Charlie's class on Buddhist ethics—all of these grow into the conditions for living with my cancer now. As Hubert Decleer, yet another one of my marvelous teachers from long ago, told me while I was studying Tibetan Buddhism in Katmandu, "It all matters. Every bit. Together these are the pieces that form a meaningful life."

Hiking through the Kiso Valley is another part of our adventures in Japan. As we set out, we first have to climb a steep hill to be rewarded with a gentle descent into a valley. It is a tough, breathless start to a four-day walking tour. My kids are concerned I won't be able to make it; I smile to reassure them. On our descent down into the valley we enter a dense, dark forest, listening to sounds of a rushing river and birdsong, the air crisp and cool, the trees sheltering us from the sun. Down and up through ravines we walk through these magical forest valleys. Occassionally we see a statue of the Jizo leaning against a tree. This is a bodhisattva of compassion, particularly associated with children, the weak and unprotected, and also travelers. As we climb up another hill, I call forward to my son, with my arms raised high, "THIS is living with cancer!"

But living with cancer also includes being overpowered by the steep hills the next day. Ben walks back and takes my small pack to carry along with his own. Rebekah takes my hand and walks by my side, singing and telling me stories and jokes in hopes of distracting me from the physical task at hand. There was no going back, and no way to our destination but to walk on. Ed takes the front, keeping the pace to move us forward. He is the one looking over his shoulder, urging us on. Despite my physical depletion, my senses urge me to take in the beauty of the place. It feels alive-alive, brimming with life, vitality, and goodness.

At an earlier time, when I was still healthy, I first sensed alive-aliveness in a forest on Maui, where I grew up (my parents had moved there when I was ten years old.) You are alive, you are dying, we are all alive, we are all dying. This is the beautiful embrace of ever-moving time. Let go!

❧

Reconciling myself to the impossibility, for now, of answering "when" I work toward feeling the value of experiencing time with a deeply felt awareness of such uncertainty. Perhaps this is one of the more notable differences between the ill and the healthy. All people might ponder this, but for most it is a theoretical question. The embodied experience of illness and decline is an opportunity to deeply feel, and thereby learn from, the impermanence of time.

My difficult goal is to surrender to it: accept the vagueness of the prognosis, instead of lashing out against it. I tell myself, "Live!" That's really the only way to orient myself in time. "Live!" Create conditions not for my own future but for others who will outlive me, particularly for my children, but hopefully, with this book, also for many people. To lay down an aspiration that will find fulfillment after I am gone.

The story of Sumedha's vow helps me reorient myself to time by inviting me in to join the crowd of people encircling Sumedha and Buddha Dipamkara. That's where I belong; not where my analytical perspective took me in past readings, where I hovered above them like an uninvited drone. Before, it was a spectacle I wanted to see and theorize about. But that distance kept me from feeling it and understanding it with my body and emotions. Once I join the crowd of men and women circling the buddha and the bodhisattva, I imagine myself standing on tiptoe, peering between heads, crouching to catch a glimpse of Dipamkara through peoples' legs, at the moment when a future time was pronounced. In his greatness and compassion, a buddha at eight feet tall is visible to everyone. The quality of a buddha's voice, sometimes called the lion's roar, makes it audible to all: "Do you see this humble ascetic lying in the mud before me? In a long distant future, he will be a buddha, the Buddha Shakyamuni." Flowers fall from the air, the earth responds with joyful rumblings, as if it is jumping up and down with glee. Rainbows fill the sky.

In the midst of my most intense and painful treatment I came to not only understand this, but to feel it: Sumedha's vow as he lay in the dirt was to create the conditions for a future in which all would be taken care of. I fall into the uncertainty of my time, falling into the mud, as it were, the mud that Sumedha dove into to cover the road for Dipamkara and his Sangha. He did it not for himself, but in order to surrender himself for the benefit of others.

To resist the uncertainty of time is to resist my opportunity to live the temporal dimension of impermanence. Falling into my uncertain future allows me to feel and learn from another dimension of my impermanence.

Again, it isn't easy. While the emotional stress of the question of "when" lessens, my everyday relationship to time is still a mess. I'm always lost in daily time. I'm constantly late to meet friends. Apologies sound hollow as they stack up into a sizable pile. Now, I thank them for their patience with me rather than asking for their forgiveness. I set all kinds of timers in my attempts at promptness, yet minutes fly by quicker than I think they will. My loss of movement in my left hand makes everyday tasks like getting dressed take just a little bit longer. It is hard to accept and adjust my calculations.

Getting lost in the eighty minutes of my lectures is particularly distressing. I set timers there too, so I'll know when we are halfway through or when I have twenty minutes left. My former, healthy self flowed through those class sessions. I instinctually sensed where we were and when we needed to speed up or slow down. Moving through discussions with that flow delighted me. As I moved around the classroom it felt something like dancing.

I miss it. I manage class times in new ways now. At first my confusion made me frantic, and I stumble when getting up to write on the white board. I learn to take a break at some point in order to recalibrate and breathe. It feels halting to me, but I see that the students benefit too. We all need to breathe. Sometimes we breathe together. I come to like this change. The first time I suggest this to my students, I refer back to a line in Gary Snyder's poem "With This Flesh" that we study in a class on Buddhist literature: "Where we breathe, we bow." When we breathe, we express gratitude by making a bow mentally or physically. As our breath moves in and out of our bodies, it is constantly changing, and thereby enabling our lives. As His Holiness the Karmapa says in his teachings, "Just by breathing we connect to all living beings."

Once, during a longer three-hour seminar, I stared at the clock not knowing if we had started one hour earlier or two. Was there another hour left to class? Two? As I tried to puzzle it out, I got more and more wound up. I had to stop. I told the students to go and take the class time to do some self-care: "Please be honest with me and yourselves. Do something good for yourselves whatever that might be. Hang out with a friend, go to the gym, take a nap, do the reading for today's class that you didn't get to yet." They smiled at me when I gave the last option in the list. When the classroom was empty, I put my head on the table and tried to figure out where I was in those three hours of class time. I headed home, relieved by knowing that my daughter's 3 p.m. school pickup would orient me to where and when I am and must be.

My illness makes me feel both lost in time and highly aware of the powerful role time has in shaping my experience in living my relationships, particularly with my children. I didn't tell them about my tumor when they were little. It didn't make sense to do so. We knew very little except that there is a tumor in my brain, and that it wasn't doing anything. How could the future make sense to them?

On that day, as we drive home from school, I tell them that they'd be with a babysitter that night because I have to go to a doctor's appointment and Dad was taking me. This is the setup for Ben, then twelve years old, to ask, "What kind of appointment?" I reply, without forethought, "They are going to take a picture of the inside of my head. There is something inside my brain that the doctor needs to see."

5. Receiving Care

In a society that places self-determination and self-sufficiency at the apex of personal development, it's hard to see oneself as dependent and in need of help. I got the message at an early age that reaching out for help would make me a burden and make people turn away from rather than toward me. This message was reinforced as I grew into adulthood: I made the choice to be a professional and a mother, and therefore it is up to me to meet the consequences and the responsibilities of that decision.

For example, the universities where I teach don't have childcare. Like so many others who are primary caretakers of their children, it's up to me to figure it out. Luckily, Bill, my most senior colleague, and chair of the department at that time, expressed nothing but delight when I told him, in the first year of my tenure-track position, that I was pregnant and would need a maternity leave in the next academic year. It is uncommon to work with people as generous as Bill. Still, I was terrified to tell him my cancer news and lay out the kind of help I would need.

Each of us feels the expectation of autonomy in our own particular ways. For me, being a mother and a professional, a motherless person, and a child from an abusive home all contributed to my reluctance to ask for help and to my wrong-headed resistance to receiving care when it is offered. It has never been a winning approach to life, but during and after my treatment it isn't possible to carry on this way. Cancer was the existential shock therapy that finally gave me another perspective on my fight against dependency.

However, giving up my long-held resistance to receiving care from others becomes necessary in my most acute times of illness. I physically have no choice but to give up my independence; I must rely upon nurses, technicians, and family to care for me. Maybe this dependency caused by my illness is something akin to being a newborn. This is terribly hard for me. My mother cared for me; she also abused me. Her own mental illness was inflicted on my tiny body. After I reached adulthood my dad shared how helpless he felt when he found bite marks on my chubby months-old legs. The mouth that made them was obviously too big to be those of my sister, who was only eighteen months older than me. It had to have been my mother who, monstrously, took my flesh into her mouth and bit down. My neurological wiring is formed in my earliest days of life to couple care together with harm.

Now, as an adult, my terminal illness gives rise to a new form of vulnerability, one that's accompanied with self-reflective dependency. Unlike a baby, I am fully aware of my needs and how others must attend to them for me. My abilities to communicate the care I need have not matured so well, yet I know that those in charge of caring for me will not intentionally harm me. In addition to the excellent, world-renowned hospitals where I receive my treatment, my loved ones will be by my side, ensuring my safety as much as they can. I have no other option, but still, it takes courage to accept my dependent condition.

My cancer gives me the opportunity to stop clinging to my illusory belief in myself as an independent being. The Karmapa has remarked that in considering life from the perspective of an independent or an interconnected person, he prefers the latter. The interconnected perspective on who we are and how we live brings greater freedom and opportunities to care for others. His teaching encourages me to put this view of myself as an interconnected individual into practice. It is hard, and I consistently fail at it. It means accepting care with grace, but it also means caring for others. I try to be aware of each failure and use it to prepare myself for how I might respond with greater help when I see a person struggling alongside me, especially another person struggling with the effects of cancer.

<hr />

For my second craniotomy, in 2017, I am only to be under twilight sedation. I have finished two years of experimental treatment, and the tumor is still growing. The surgeons will need me to come in and out of consciousness in order to ask me to move parts of the left side of my body. The surgeon is going after the part of the tumor closest to the motor strip on the right side of my brain. He wants to remove all of it this time—rather than leave some like they did back in 2014—but he doesn't want to paralyze me. It is the same challenge surgeons faced in 2002 and 2014. The idea that I will be somewhat awake after my skull had been sawed through, knowing the surgeon is delicately cutting away parts of my brain, is crazy to me.

I describe it all to Karmapa when I receive time to speak with him privately in Delhi at the book launch for *Interconnected* a few months before the surgery. Sitting before him, with Damcho by my side, he pays careful attention as he always does. Following his moments of internal quiet and stillness, he opens his eyes and gently tells me, "It won't be so bad." This doesn't feel like a formulaic, dismissive response. He shares what he confidently knows. Then he repeats it in terms that are more common: "It's like one of those things that seem like they'll be really bad before they happen, but afterward aren't really so bad." I get that. OK, good. I believe him, I believe in him. I keep the Karmapa's reassurance close to me and draw my memories of my time with him, and those of my most happy "alive-alive" experiences with my family, around me like a shawl that encircles me through the coming hard months.

In order to receive care from others I had to learn how to express the kind of help I needed and the form in which I would be most able to receive it. This layer of knowing my needs and expressing them to others was hard to master, but as I practiced, I was sometimes surprised to find that I was getting good at it. I was proud of myself when, in the moments before my second craniotomy, I directed the famous surgeon Dr. B to see me in my fullness as a person and not only a malignant tumor.

Like with the period leading up to my first craniotomy, the pace of events picked up rapidly before my second. My first significant seizure prepared me for the news that the tumor had changed. For the first time in all these dozens of MRIs when they injected the contrasting dye into me, I light up. This shows that the cancer is more aggressive. The 10 percent of the tumor that the excellent surgeon in 2014 felt she couldn't reasonably remove without a high degree of causing harm now must be removed. Ed and I consult with the surgeon who performed the first craniotomy. She doesn't want to do this second surgery. We turn to the doctors who had overseen my care during the experimental chemotherapy trial at UCSF. One of the oncologists tells me she'd put my case in front of the chief neurosurgeon, Dr. B. She was confident he could and would do the surgery.

Ed phones a world-renowned neuro-oncologist at Duke University. A friend of a friend had connected us to him. Replaying the conversation for me later, Ed mimicked the accent and good-but-gruff spirit of my great-uncle Julie, a loving, tough, Jewish lawyer who spent his life in Brooklyn, and who had stepped up as a surrogate father to my dad after his father had died. Ed first thanked the Duke doctor for talking with him and got back, "No thanks needed! This is what I do." This is what people in relationships do: they take care of one another. When I reflect upon the past, I see the layers of care are as thick as the layers of abuse and fear. Ed described my medical history and the immediate decision facing us of doing the second surgery.

"What's the problem? You got Dr. B? You do the surgery! No question!" His impatient certainty was a gift. Our deliberation was done for us with this phone call. Ed asked, "Can we make a donation to a charity you support to thank you for your consultation?" "No! This is my work. This is how I help people. OK?!" His words were emphasized with a cranky compassion.

I don't travel up to San Francisco for a consultation with Dr. B, this demi-god of the brain cancer realm. The trip feels like too much for me. A phone consult has to do. I am scared to talk to him. Scared of all of this.

Ed and I prepare a list of questions we are going to ask him together. My plan is to hide out behind Ed's deep voice. But the surgeon calls when Ed is at his office and unreachable. I breathe deeply and plunge into our questions by myself. Dr. B is kind and patient, answering each question clearly and then asking if I understood. When I reach the final question, I conclude with "That's it." "Anything else?" he asks, inviting me to go on. "Um." I consider it and then ask, "Are there questions I haven't asked but I should?" "No. You did a good job; you asked good questions."

I finish our phone call with my decision: "I want to do the surgery." "Good." He affirms my conclusion.

Ten days later I am in pre-op, lying on a gurney in a hospital gown. A nurse writes B's name on the right side of my forehead. For the next six to eight hours my brain is his. Great attention is taken to ensure no mistakes are made on what part of my brain is being removed. That's good.

First, I speak with the anesthesiologist resident. "How are you?" he asks. "I'm scared," I say quietly. All of my motions and speech feel small and muted. I'm hiding inside myself. He nods and replies with an empathetic smile that communicates, "Of course you are."

I take a breath and tell him the details of my particular concerns: "I had this twilight sedation with my first surgery, a biopsy, fifteen years ago. It was the most hellish experience of my life."

His eyes fill with concern. "Walk me through it. Tell me what happened."

I narrate my experience at Mass General in 2002: The chief anesthesiologist came into the pre-op and barked at his resident: "She's young and healthy. Give her the minimum necessary." There was no topical numbing, no valium or other drug to put me in some kind of fuzzy state before four shots of local anesthetic went into my head and they screwed in the titanium frame that would stabilize it for the surgery. The pain was so intense I was simultaneously on the verge of passing out and throwing up. One nurse had to rush over with oxygen, another with a container for my vomit. I heard a saw removing a piece of my skull, felt pulling sensations as they cut into my brain and a tugging as it was sewn back up. I heard the surgeon shouting: "No! Not there!" I was in and out of consciousness for seven or eight hours. They had promised a drug that would make me forget the experience, but, it seems, they didn't give it to me.

The anesthesiologist for this third brain surgery listens to my first go-round intently and waited until I was finished with my list of torments. He sees it the same way: "That is horrible. Really horrible. We won't let that happen to you. I promise you."

I feel trust. I believe him. He won't let that happen to me.

I meet Dr. B for the first time soon after, when he joins the team of two surgeons, two anesthesiologists, and two surgical nurses, all now encircling me. Ed stands by my side. Dr. B talks us through the surgery: how they will bring me back to a twilight state of consciousness several times to instruct me to move a limb, test my visual tracking, or answer some questions. He promises they will bring me back as briefly as possible. "We need to do this so we protect your brain functions." I nod. He asks us, "Any other questions?" I looked at Ed, then back at Dr. B.

I don't have any other questions, but without any forethought I find myself saying, "No. But if it's OK, I'd like to tell you a few things about myself. Is that OK?" "Yes," he replies, free of any sign of irritation. I remember his eyes holding mine. "I'm a mother: my kids are still at home. I have a daughter who is fourteen and a son almost seventeen. They need me. I'm also a university professor and a scholar. I've spent my life cultivating my mind." When I pause, Dr. B says, "You have an accomplished life." "That's not it." I correct what I want to communicate: "I have a full life and I need to live it. I want you to know that." He nods, showing he understands.

As the residents wheel me off to the OR and away from Ed, I wish my love a good day. The residents chuckle. Was it because they think, "How could he possibly have a good day?" Or that in the face of what I was about to experience, my concern is for him. Lying on the gurney I still cling to my role as caretaker, not the one being cared for.

A few times during the surgery I hear Dr. B say, "Karen, we need you to move your left foot, can you do that for us?" I move it. "You are doing really great," he offers compassionately. "How many fingers do you see?" "Two." "Excellent. Everything is going well."

His voice is soothing and protective. I move in and out of consciousness like drifting in the air. At one point the sensation is smashed by a sudden downwind when I hear Dr. B say in a loud, direct, and forceful voice, "Get her blood pressure down! Now!"

A voice responds, "It's fine; it's not that high compared to where it's been."

Dr. B's thunderclap again: "Get it down! NOW!" then an acquiescent "Yes, sir!"

However long later, my eyes are open as I'm wheeled away from the OR. "You are doing amazingly well," both residents reassure me. Again, there is delight in their voices.

Then this exchange. I hear my voice, calm and quiet: "Can I ask a question? Why was Dr. B focused on my blood pressure at the end?"

Surgery resident: "When we need to close an area that has been previously opened and sutured, there can be more blood than usual, making it challenging to do. With a lower blood pressure, less blood, better suturing."

The anesthesiologist resident follows: "You were never in danger. Your blood pressure wasn't threatening you."

Whoever: "Wow! You are observant. It's kind of incredible you picked up on that."

Yes, I am observant. As a reader, I've been training to be observant for a long time.

After the surgery I need help with my smallest and most personal bodily functions. My sense of self as an independent, self-sufficient being is gone in less than a day. With remarkable skills my nurse offers intimate care with respect and with the awareness that my personal boundaries are rapidly shifting. Peeing is a complicated series of actions of getting to a commode from my hospital bed and completing the act in front of others; I am not allowed to be left alone, not for a single second. When I can't make my bladder empty, my ICU nurse asks, "How about we try the sleepover prank of putting your hand in water? That works for some people." "Sure, why not?" Remarkably, it works.

Once, on the way back to my hospital bed, my oversized sock entangles with the commode stand and the whole thing almost toppled over. Ed and the nurse rush to keep me upright. My now fully exposed bottom is the least of my concerns. "Oh man, if you had fallen, Dr. B would have had me fired, no doubt," my new nurse friend lets out once I'm back in bed.

"Sorry?" I say.

"Oh, you're good. Everything OK?"

"Is Dr. B scary?" I ask.

"To the nurses, yeah. But it's only because he wants the very best for his patients. He is ferocious for his patients." Dr. B has been consistently gentle with me, no arrogance, only concern. The ferocity experienced by the staff is a form of care toward me

My nurses each nurture me in their own style in relationship to my quickly evolving needs. One nurse who cares for me after surgery in the ICU is maternal, while another is conspiratorial, rolling his eyes at the arduous protocol of care my surgeon had ordered even as he acknowledges that Dr. B would accept no less than the best level of care for his patients. When I tell another nurse that I'm scared of the MRI I will soon undergo, she winks at me and gives me a pill to soothe my anxiety. "Chew it up real fast," she tells me with a wink. "Rock and roll, sister," she calls after me as the attendant wheels me to my MRI.

These people were sensitive observers and good listeners. In my healthy life the challenge is knowing and signaling what my needs are. Being honest is much easier in my vulnerable state when I am not calculating people's reactions to my requests for care: How much would this cost me? Would living interconnected with me drain them of vitality for the future?

In the moments after the surgery, I desperately want water; it had been a day or more since I'd been allowed to drink anything, and it is forbidden still. My ICU nurse places drops of water in my mouth with a kind of lollipop-sponge that I suck at. I feel like a nursing newborn pursing my lips to indicate my need. Over and over, she makes this simple but significant movement of care by refilling the sponge with water and placing it in my mouth. I won't be allowed to care for myself for a few days, not even in the smallest ways.

⸎

All people are indeed our mothers, time and time again. My serious illness makes this Buddhist teaching come alive. According to traditional Theravada Buddhist descriptions of our universe, its central point, Mount Meru, is surrounded by four continents in each of the cardinal directions. Life differs greatly on each of these continents. On Uttarakuru, the northern continent, all babies can be nursed by any grownup, whose fingers are a kind of milk dispenser. When a person encounters a hungry baby, they simply place a finger in the baby's mouth and milk flows into that suckling. On Uttarakuru, all people can fill the mothering role in this most elemental kind of way. In this imagined land, all people can and do provide the necessary condition for life for any other person, especially those who are the most dependent and helpless. Uttarakuru is a part of our world and yet set apart from us.

In our world, people can't or don't care for each other with this kind of attention to need and fluidity of action. While biologically fantastic, this brief description of an imagined place describes a human community of endless relational possibilities. Any person can step into the role of nursing mother and then, I suppose, step out of it. It invites me to envision a boundless human capacity to nurture any other person realized into action. It takes an ethical ideal—all people are our mothers—and then imagines how that might work in embodied practice.

I recently told this story to a woman I sat next to at a fundraising dinner. This cosmological story jumped into my head when she told me she was a dietician for critically ill people. Her work is to make the right mixtures of nutrients that an individual needs for their recovery. She also determines the best pathways to feed her patients: IVs, portals, feeding tubes, etc.

I hesitated before telling this story of the world from another time and culture to someone I'd just met. Maybe it's too strange and she would look around for another place to sit? However, that wasn't her reaction; not at all. She stepped right into this brief story, and her eyes filled with tears. She saw herself as filling this role. "This is a lot like what I do," she told me, confirming the connection I saw between her professional actions and those in the story. We were two grown, independent, accomplished women, and we were strangers. In this shared moment we each found our place in this vision of a world of ever-present care. Perhaps she had never thought of her work from that broader perspective; I hadn't really seen the connections between this story and the many ways people are acting out its ethic in the world around us.

This brief, serendipitous conversation inspired me to move around inside this story. My impulse is to place myself into it as the person with something to give in order to nurture a person in need. Just a few months before, I took a friend's baby into my arms so she could eat her lunch before delivering a paper at a conference. Her baby needed to nurse, his mother needed to feed herself. Rocking him back and forth, I put a finger in his mouth to soothe him. He sucked at it so vigorously it felt like my finger was caught up in a vacuum. He sucked away, calmed until he could be totally fulfilled by his mother's milk. I am like the mother, and I am also like the baby in need of care. In the legend of Uttarakuru, caring for another is natural and not burdensome. Can you imagine living in a world where exposing our need for care and offering care is as natural and responsive as this?

As far as I know, the descriptions of this place don't tell us what happens after a baby is cared for in this communal fashion; there is nothing in the one brief story I know. It leaves me curious—what happens next?

In the midst of the agony of disease and treatment, the comforting presence of loved ones—be it a parent, partner, teacher, friend, or buddha—provides a continuity of care that enables a suffering person to move into their future. I will be cared for beyond the hours of a nurse's shift, for my entire stay in the hospital, and when I move back into my home and ordinary life.

My father and sister respond to the escalation of my disease and prolonged need for care with generous offers to put their own lives on hold and come to my home to help. My relationship with both of them has at times been complicated. We shared the reality of my mother's death but had very different experiences and memories of my mother's abuse. My anger at my father lasted for many years, as did my anger and distrust toward my sister.

These feelings greatly saddened my dad, and me too. While my love for him compelled me to make space for his assessments of what took place during my teenage years, I was often unkind in clinging to my own interpretation of my childhood trauma. I felt that I had been left alone and unprotected. I failed to see the lack of resources he had at the time of my mother's abuse and how challenging it was to suddenly be a single parent to two teenage girls while he was trying to put his life back together. My sister's skeletal memories of our childhood added another obstacle to our emotional processing.

Unlike her, I hold vivid memories of my early childhood and the many ways my mother abused us. I can still see us all in the

kitchen, my father urging my sister to give my mom a reconciling hug after a day of screaming and who knows what else.
As soon as my sister is in striking distance my mom lashes out,
punching her in the face. My dad springs at my mom, holding
her arms and taking her away from his children.

Still, he leaves us with her when they separate for a time, I
imagine because he didn't know what else to do, and perhaps in
order to preserve his own well-being. After the separation my
sister and I live with my mom, but we see my dad almost daily.
My sister, older and bigger than me, fills the role of my protector
many times. By the time we were teens she has grown bigger
than my petite mom. One time when my mom lashes out at me
physically after a verbal assault, my sister places herself in front
of me. As I remember it, she tells our mom, "If you hurt either
one of us again, I'll fight back."

Yet, when my mom dies, my sister is just enough older than
me that she has other places to go and friends to be with. She's
out of the house a lot, as is my dad, and I am often left alone
for long periods of time. I feel abandoned and afraid. No one's
protecting me from the many forms of fear that prey upon me
late at night, jumping at every sound I hear in our empty house.
Filling the sudden void in our family dynamic, my sister and I
fight often. We hurt each other, physically and verbally. She who
was my protector as a girl now becomes an assailant. One brutal
evening while driving erratically on a windy, rural road—much
like the one my mom drove on when she got into her fatal accident—she blames me for my mother's death. It triggers a panic
attack.

My sister tells me I was the cause of much of my mom's bru-
tality. She hates me.

The trauma of my childhood abuse and the clarity of my

memories lie beneath the surface of my relationship with both my father and my sister, and these things sometimes rupture into our adult lives in ways that are painful. We always remain a family, managing the destructive emotions that arise as best we can, most often by not seeing each other too frequently.

All of this makes me a little wary of my dad's offer to stay for a month in 2017 during my post-surgery treatment of simultaneous radiation and chemotherapy. I live with the commitment I make to myself, heard and acknowledged by the Karmapa, to be oriented by love rather than fear. It gives me courage to turn toward my dad and receive his care. Without the Karmapa's teachings on the ways in which impermanence gifts us the opportunities to become new people and reform relationships, I'm not sure I would be able to make that choice.

The radiologist tells us that the first month of the daily treatment will be OK, but that by the last three and a half weeks I will be exhausted and in need of intensive assistance, especially in driving to my sessions. I accept my dad's offer. This all happens about the same time as his eightieth birthday and not long after his surgery for heart disease. Time isn't unfolding as it should. He is caring for his ill daughter instead of the other way around.

Day after day he wakes up before his grandkids to ready their breakfasts and drive them to school. Day after day he then takes me to my radiation appointments. Holding my hands, he sighs when I am called back for my turn with the radiation machine. As usual, I offer him my forehead for a kiss. When I come out of the radiation room, he holds out a drink to cover the bad taste in my mouth and to manage my low-grade nausea.

The tech staff all come to know and like him; they relay his messages to me if he's in the restroom when I come out from my treatment. Otherwise he is right outside the entrance to the treatment area with that same pained face. He'd say, "You OK? Let's get you home."

He stays with my family until the end of my treatment. On one of our slow walks with my dog around our neighborhood, I thanked him for all he was doing for me. "You are a good dad. I'm grateful." I know he has wanted to hear those words from me for a very long time. I also know that this is the first time in a very long while that I can say them in a way that feels true to me, in a way that feels right in my mind, body, and heart. I am honestly grateful to my illness for creating these conditions for this change in my relationship with my dad. This deep love is my silver lining, though it has come at quite a cost.

In the midst of those weeks, my sister also flies across the country to be with us. Our relationship is still complicated. As adults, I was the one resistant to healing. I wouldn't let go of the pain and anger that formed, layer upon layer, between us. I tightly grasped my mistrust. I didn't think I'd find anything that would pry it away. After my first craniotomy in 2014, my sister had offered to come care for me. "No. No. Thanks," I say, "but no. We'll be fine with our friends' help."

I still have work to do to put down my anger and fear. I wish I could sit down next to the venerable nun Kisa Gotami and ask her what to do. She found a way to put down the intense suffering of her child dying; surely, I could put down the anger clenched in my hardened heart. Receiving my dad's tender care in those first weeks gave me the courage to accept my sister's offer. It gave me the space to acknowledge the respect I feel for her willingness to offer her help again after my rejection of her three years earlier.

During her stay, she comforts me in a particular way that I can't name, but I can describe how the moments feel. One day after radiation treatment she and I are in the room in my home where she is sleeping. Lying face-to-face on the bed, she reaches out and interlaces her fingers with mine. I cry deeply, the tears surfacing from the depths of a deep, deep well of trauma and loss. She stays with me as I cry and she begins crying too. "I don't want to die. I don't want to leave them," I tell her.

"I know," she says.

"How can this be happening again?" I ask her. She knows just what I am referring to: our difficult motherless years of growing into adulthood. We each had to find our own way on our paths, yet there is still a bond between us unlike any other. Although we had trampled upon it for years, its strength is returning. We cry and cry, our faces are red, gasping for air with occasional sobs. Only with her can I let out my suffering like this. She holds my hand until I am ready to stop.

In our formative years she was my companion in trauma and death, if not always in a caring way. And although we rarely talk about our abuse, and she doesn't remember it with the clarity that I do, I know in this moment of surviving this new trauma of my disease and the pummeling treatment, she feels it alongside me. With her I can feel this pain and get it out of my body.

Trusting that I'll always be cared for scares me. What if my illness becomes so disgusting or I become such a burden that I will no longer receive care? I fear that in some unknown, approaching future my disease will progress in ways that make it more visible, dramatic, and unpalatable. What if my temperament or emotions change and it becomes too difficult to care for me? What if I lose cognitive abilities or basic bodily functions? As much as I feel myself changing—lacking strength, forgetting words, falling into a state of woozy, groggy focus—I still write "what if" instead of "when." These are no longer conditional questions. When that time begins, and I become increasingly vulnerable, I must maintain the courage to ask for and receive care.

The Pali canon includes stories of when the Buddha and his attendant, Ananda, are the only ones willing to physically care for monks who are so sick that they are abandoned by their companion monks. One story from the *Mahavastu* tells of one such monk. The Buddha himself tends to the monk's soiled body with his own hands, as he ministers to the monk's distressed mind by teaching the Dharma. As translated by Thanissaro Bhikkhu:

> Then the Blessed One addressed Ven. Ananda: "Go fetch some water, Ananda. We will wash this monk."
>
> "As you say, lord," Ven. Ananda replied, and he fetched some water. The Blessed One sprinkled water on the monk, and Ven. Ananda washed him off. Then—with the Blessed One taking the monk by the head, and Ven. Ananda taking him by the feet—they lifted him up and placed him on a bed.
>
> Then the Blessed One, from this cause, because of this event, had the monks assembled and asked them, "Is there a sick monk in that dwelling over there?"
>
> "Yes, O Blessed One, there is."
>
> "And what is his sickness?"
>
> "He has dysentery, O Blessed One."
>
> "But does he have an attendant?"
>
> "No, O Blessed One."
>
> "Then why don't the monks attend to him?"
>
> "He doesn't do anything for the monks, lord, which is why they don't attend to him."

"Monks, you have no mother, you have no father, who might tend to you. If you don't tend to one another, who then will tend to you? Whoever would tend to me should tend to the sick.

The Buddha then goes on to enumerate five qualities of a good caregiver and five qualities of a good care receiver, as well as five qualities of a poor caregiver and five qualities of a poor patient. Among them, competency and compassion are two you would expect of the good caregiver, while the patient is expected to be obedient and honest in admitting their needs.

The seriously ill of today might all too easily relate to that sick, abandoned monk. The desperation or isolation depicted in the story is perhaps not that different from those who struggle with the denial of care by insurance companies or the disappearance of family or friends who can't or don't know how to take care of them. Our results-oriented society equates caring with fixing, and some conditions have no fix. For me, when I am at my worst, what I really need is for those who love me to see what is happening to me. My good health shifts to fragility, and my strength to vulnerability. I feel that they can't do anything to fix me, but they can see me. I need care, just as we all do: in our natural state since birth, in our interconnected lives in adulthood, and in our shifting lives of dependence as we grow ill and old. The Buddha is a model of both receiving and giving care. The Buddha gave the opportunity to care for him, not only to Ananda, his personal attendant who cared for his bodily needs, but also to his lay patrons and his Sangha. The Buddha, we're often told, was capable of great miracles and so didn't really need this care. But he offered the opportunity for others to take responsibility of his well-being as a means of earning merit, i.e., good karma. A buddha is the greatest field of merit, and caring for them is said to earn one enormous rewards.

I am scared that a time will come when I become so sick I will no longer receive the care I need because my caregivers may worry that the treatment could do more harm than good. Some surgeons shied from doing my brain surgery because the risk of paralysis, to their minds, outweighed the possibility that the surgery would do me any good. On a smaller scale, friends and family talk about seemingly anything other than my cancer for fear of saying the wrong thing and hurting my feelings. People with sickness are abandoned routinely in all sorts of ways. Left alone, rendered voiceless, pushed out of sight by insurance companies that refuse treatment.

I am incredibly privileged. Our health insurance is good; during one phone conversation with an insurance agent, my husband was told that the agent had never seen a policy as good as ours.

And yet, there is a medication that is curing people with a different form of cancer but the same genetic mutation as I have. This drug is approved by the FDA for this other cancer but not for the kind I carry around in my head. This means that there is a likely cure for my cancer, but my oncologist cannot prescribe it to me because it would be for an off-label use, which our insurance would not cover. As he told me, he'd write a prescription for me today, but it would cost my family upward of $10,000 a month, perhaps many multiples of that number. The three of us look at each other with frustration, disbelief, longing. It's the "millionaires' cure," Dr. Lai says. "We'll get to FDA approval." He's determined. I'm determined to hold on until we reach that point.

Thus, as privileged as I am, there are treatments that are out of my reach, just as the treatment I do receive is beyond the reach of so many others. I commit myself to being oriented by love as I live with my cancer. If I am to live by that commitment, I need to concern myself with others who also carry my form of cancer, people who aren't as privileged as I am: those who don't have access to the best doctors, to the medicines we must take, to the insurance to pay for it all. How do I do this? It is a question I carry with me daily. Even when there are small opportunities to act, I fail.

The very last day of radiation, I feel relief as my dad pulls up to the hospital. Like all other days, I internally make the aspiration that all people inside this building feel an alleviation of suffering and heightened happiness. If I can contribute to that shift, let me do so. I am met at the nuclear medicine area with congratulations; I'd made it to this finish line! After this session today the brain radiation is done for good. My brain has been radiated to the limit. Here is one fixed piece of time. This is the day I cross a form of treatment off the list. I have to get through it and then it is done. The technologist apologizes because my appointment is delayed: "We have a pediatric case coming in after you today. It is quite complicated to set up for a little guy."

"Oh! It's not all about me!" I scold myself again. My suffering under the radiation machine is ending, but the device will keep moving around other people's heads—children's heads, destroying cells in a part of their bodies in order to prolong their young lives. "Oh!" As I lie on the metal table and feel my face mask snapping me onto it to keep me absolutely still, my mantras begin spontaneously moving from the crown of my head down through my feet. Karmapa Khyenno, Karmapa, think of me. And please be with this little person too. I imagine the boy who will soon lay where I am. I visualize him resting on top of my body, my arms encircling him, helping him stay still. Karmapa Khyenno. Karmapa remember this child. Please, be with this child.

As soon as I am free from my mask and the metal exam table, I see the foam they've cut up to encircle the next patient, the child who will lay on the cold metal table from which I just got up. My dad greets me outside the radiation area with a huge smile. "You are through the radiation! You did it!" I did. I feel deep relief, even while knowing that the side effects will go on for at least another year, or I don't know, maybe years.

There is a woman inside the elevator when we get on. With just a quick glance I notice her glassy eyes and little else except the sounds of her sniffling. I cram myself into a corner with my head as far away as possible; I am terrified that I'll catch the flu that's going around. Then she speaks: "My son is having radiation right now. He's only two, he's having seizures. This is what the doctors say to do."

Moving into the open, I speak directly to her face. "I am so sorry, I am so very sorry." What else is there to say? "What is his name?" I ask.

"R-Jon."

"R-Jon, R-Jon," I repeat out loud as we reach the lobby: "Is it OK if I say a prayer for R-Jon? Will that be OK?"

"Yes." My method of prayer is likely not what she imagines, but it feels OK.

As we move toward the lobby she asks if I know how to get to the cafeteria. I point the way and repeat that I will pray for R-Jon.

As my dad turns the car out of the hospital complex, I crumble. I get through seven weeks of radiation appointments, but all I feel is the last few moments. I failed! I FAILED! I didn't ask if she had anyone to wait with her. I could easily have done that. Why didn't I offer to get her something to eat? What the fuck, Karen? Easing other's suffering? Fail! Mother of R-Jon, I'm sorry!

I call Charlie, as I often do when the intensity of my physical and emotional pain crushes me. I tell him what happened. He listens deeply, as he always does. There is silence on the phone for a brief moment. "Karen, you did do something. You made the wish, and you recognize you couldn't fulfill it. You can use this to learn for next time."

My friends who helped Ed and me over the previous two months, who provided much of the care we needed to live through my intense treatments, gather that night at our house for a champagne toast to mark the end of my months of concurrent radiation and chemotherapy. My family is encircled by these loving, generous friends as we all stand around our dining room table, a place where we have shared meals and companionship over many years. I feel loved, cared for. I feel their generosity. There are many toasts, and my loved ones praise me for my courage.

I want to tell them about R-Jon and his mother. It feels selfish to do that, in the midst of this celebration my friends are eager to share with me, a celebration of their kindness as much as my survival. But I can't hold off my tears.

As they hold glasses to toast the hopefully easier days ahead, I thank them for all they do to help my family. And then, I tell them that I am a failure. I'm not the courageous person they believe me to be. I fail at caring for others while I receive my own care. I have to tell them. I can't stop myself. Their generosity grows larger still as they listen to me describe meeting R-Jon's mom and how much care she needed, and how I failed

to act. Some of them cry too. I thank them for their companionship and how my experience today made me feel the reality that
many, many people don't have a community like I do.

I have felt something I might name as shame for having cancer.
For many years I told very few people about my tumor and the
likelihood of its progression into cancer. I didn't want people to
pity me or, scarier still, to be wary of me. Susan Sontag argues
in her landmark essay, *Illness as Metaphor*, that illness has long
been equated with weakness, and cancer is seen as a symbol for
something out of control. This resonates. As an abused person
I have long sought to conceal the many ways in which loss of
control has characterized my life. A lack of restraint even in my
brain cells felt like a failure of sorts.

Sometimes, after reflection, I do reveal that I have brain cancer. I struggle with the question of whether I should tell my
students. I do in cases when I will be less authentically present
with them if I were to try to hide it.

My closest friends step in and organize help on my and Ed's
behalf. They create a space that brings together people whose
only connections previously were through me. I become a hub
in a new community. Kelly takes over organizing food by setting
up a calendar for people to sign up to bring a meal; Kim and
Steve coordinate rides for our kids to school and to activities.
Knowing me and my deficiencies well, they set up parameters
for caregivers: "When you drop off food or kids at the house,
Karen will invite you in. Do not accept. If she begs you to come
in, do not accept her offer to get you something to eat or drink!
Don't stay, even if she insists, but if you lose that one, don't stay
more than five minutes."

While it was humorous at the time, and all my dear ones

got these inside jokes, it wasn't really necessary. It's important for me not to be dismissive about how sick I am. Most often friends are cautious about disturbing whatever ebb or flow is happening on a particular day, and I can hardly rouse myself to notice that there was some activity in the house. I am not getting the door, even if I hear the bell. At most, I am often only conscious of distant sounds of companionship, like I remember from childhood when I fell asleep to the talk and laughter of my parents and their friends at one of my mom's lovely dinner parties.

These are the comforting sounds of presence; I wasn't alone. That condition gives rise to gratitude I'm not alone, but that isn't to say that I am not lonely. People almost always tell me I look good. Offered in kindness, it makes me feel isolated and alone in my experience; I know better, and I need them to acknowledge what is happening. I stop wearing any makeup on my down days when I want to be seen as I am. When the large dark circles around my eyes are clearly visible, I don't look so good. I encourage my dearest friends to tell me truthfully how I look: Kelly tells me I look gaunt and tells me to get the most caloric item on the lunch menu, agrees that my short hair, after radiation took most of it, is not my best look; I'm a long-hair person. Steve can see when I hit the wall of exhaustion and encourages me to go get my nap, offering to pick up Rebekah from school if it'll let me sleep longer.

But it is hard for all my loved ones to look clearly into the uncertainty of diagnosis and prognosis with me. I understand the impulse to take comfort by focusing on the positive possibilities that the worst won't happen to me, that I'll have longer to live than the statistics show. Statistics aren't determinative. They are not a prediction of the future.

My few friends who have been through their own cancer treatment, and those I've met through their memoirs, can understand my embodied experience from the inside. They have been my guide to accepting care with a modicum of graciousness. I talk to my friend Rebecca, who survived cancer in her early thirties, about my discomfort with receiving help from others; everyone has a full plate and now my friends have to provide this care for me too. Her response became a great teaching on interconnectedness for me: "We don't have to do these things—we get to do these things." This simple shift in words, from "have to" to "get to" emphasizes that our responsibility for one another is an opportunity to experience interconnection. There are links to one another that shine when impermanence changes our conditions.

I have a lot to learn from my memories of my son as a toddler on the verge of being completely toilet trained. The missing piece was his resistance to sitting on the toilet to poo. He developed his own system: he would go into the bathroom and ask me to put him in a diaper and then leave and shut the door behind me. A minute later he would call to me that he was done and needed the diaper taken off. In I went, flushed the poo down the toilet, cleaned his bottom, after which he happily put his underwear back on. It was an amazing arrangement to me, one of his own design, that built up his courage toward self-sufficiency. I love how he directed my care just as he needed it.

For me, facing my fear that I am dependent on others takes courage. The Karmapa teaches me that I'll find courage when I allow myself to authentically feel my vulnerability as an interconnected person. Moving past self-care as an adult brings an opportunity for a new form of courage: the courage to feel one's own impermanence, to feel one's dependence and connection to others. Sometimes, people we count on will let us down. It is inevitable; it is survivable. There will be other forms of care.

⚜

As my experience of receiving care changes, it leads me to new companions who are also sources of attention and comfort, including our dog Biz, whose footsteps now clack on the wood floor as I type. If I were writing on an old-fashioned typewriter, rather than my computer keyboard, we might make some kind of melody.

I grew up without pets. My parents had no connection to animals, given their New York City upbringing. Over the years my students tried to convince me to get my kids a pet, and we do eventually adopt an old dog, Biz, brought to us by friends when they no longer have the best conditions for his happiness. Elderly and sweet, we become his retirement family.

The rest of the story follows the usual patterns: Biz quickly becomes my dog. I walk him daily, feed him, and spend time with him as promises from the rest of my family to do those tasks are forgotten as soon as he settles into our home, just as I knew they would.

When I sleep for hours every day following my surgery, Biz sits by my bed, looking at me with eyes I anthropomorphize into looks of concern and love. Caring for him makes me care for myself; his walks get me moving every morning, and the simple chore of feeding him makes me get out of bed. Most importantly, these tasks remind me that even in my weakest state I can care for others, an essential condition for feeling alive. It wasn't all blissful coexistence: his geriatric bad breath and farts bring on my nausea, and I have to shut him away from me when I attempt to steady myself.

There is something about being with Biz that is unlike any other companion. His silent attentiveness requests me to just be with him; his basic needs have been met. For many people seeing animals as sources of nurture is almost a given. It was a surprise for me. With Biz by my side, not only was I literally not alone—I also felt less lonely.

I've read many ill people's descriptions of the space between physical solitude and emotional isolation. One of my favorite Buddhist stories prepares me to receive Biz's capacity for care: the story of the elephant Parileyaka.

This story begins with the problems of human society. The monks living around the Buddha are quarreling about this and that. Even after the Buddha corrects their behavior several times, the monks' conflicts continue. They have fallen into self-ishness and disregard for the welfare of their companions. The Buddha goes to a forest by himself, leaving them on their own to find their way back to correct living in community. In the forest, it may appear that the Buddha has isolated himself from social dynamics, but there he encounters a majestic elephant king named Parileyaka. This elephant came to the forest due to circumstances parallel to those that bring the Buddha there: his herd resisted his teachings on how to solve disharmony among them, and the elephant king left them on their own to repair their society and reestablish tranquility.

Parileyaka takes up this most precious opportunity to care for the Buddha, gathering fruit for his meal, warming water for his bath, creating a bed for him in the forest, and sweeping his living space with a branch he holds in his trunk.

After some time and admonishment by the larger society

around them, both the monastic Sangha and the elephant herd correct their ways and go in search of their leaders. Human and animal communities arrive at the same time to see Parileyaka's daily routine of care and the Buddha's gracious acceptance of it. Living in relationships of care is always possible—and always necessary for living.

In a curious subplot we are reminded that death is ever-present too—not because of a lack of care, but because death is a part of reality. A monkey is the first to witness Parileyaka's service to the Buddha. Inspired, she finds a way to make her own offering by collecting a honeycomb. At first the Buddha leaves it untouched, as eating the comb would harm the insects inside. Understanding what must be done, the monkey carefully removes each insect with a twig before placing it again before Buddha, who now receives it.

The monkey's joy at giving this gift propels her into movement. She springs through the trees, dancing high above the forest floor. The monkey fills the sky with joy until she falls and lands on an arrow-sharp branch and dies. This is not the end of the monkey's story. She is reborn in one of the heavenly realms, bringing her one step closer to a future human birth and the possibility of awakening. Her death is thus used to teach us that the Buddha is indeed the most powerful field of growing one's own merit, but the lesson is there for all of us: caring for others is vital for our future well-being, and accepting care from others is a form of kindness.

In working to overcome my vulnerability to receiving care, I hopefully give my loved ones an opportunity to develop something in themselves as well. It is not for me to name what those virtues or experiences might be. Some tell me they feel good in being a source of strength or kindness, or in facing their own fears. Yes, I also find that many people don't want to know about my illness. I can sense that knowing my diagnosis/prognosis is too much. It hurts, but I understand. Talking about my cancer is to ask people to come with me into the intimate, frightening space of death—mine and, someday, theirs too. In these cases I usually back off right away. With my most beloved people, though, I learn to press on, asking for them to be with me in this.

It is extremely hard to learn how to talk about death—my death or anyone's. It is not only an unfamiliar topic, but a different way of speaking. We are learning together how to communicate about decline and loss, about the truth of impermanence and how to speak about it, to listen to it. How to ask and answer questions when the inevitability of loss is resisted in so many ways.

⚬⚬⚬

Growing up on the island of Maui, beauty is always around me. I don't take it for granted. I learn in my teenage years how to let it seep into me to counterbalance the loneliness and pain I feel after my mom died. I can finally express a realization I had as a girl, which had been somewhere between conscious and subconscious awareness: if there is so much beauty in the world, there must be more than suffering.

The views of the ocean, the mountains, the shifting clouds, or the smell of wild ginger inspire hope. Stay inspired, I tell myself now. Sometimes I find it almost impossible, and the best I can do is repeat that to myself. If there is so much beauty in the world, there must be more than suffering. This becomes my self-fashioned mantra, and "Karmapa Khyenno" almost always follows.

Being cared for by beauty in its nonsentient forms relies upon cultivating my sense perception in new ways. Natural beauty reaches out to me, but it isn't easy to feel held by a mountain or strengthened by the ocean, accompanied by a sea turtle who holds our gaze as we swim through shared waves.

I don't want to be saccharine or overly romantic about this. I've found that I can participate in natural beauty when I'm open to experiencing a different kind of agency. Dogen, the twelfth-century Zen master, in his masterful *Shobogenzo*, wrote, "The blue mountains constantly walking." I can't explain to myself what this means. I know when I sit in the long pasture grasses moving on the hillsides formed by erosion on majestic Mount Haleakala, it feels like I'm sitting in the lap of the Buddha.

The year following my third brain surgery, in 2017, is full of trauma. During my recovery from brain surgery and the start of radiation and chemotherapy, my husband's mother dies. It is a huge loss for all of us. Following closely after that, my son's twenty-four-year-old mentor dies in a motorcycle accident in front of Ben's school. It is a shocking death of someone who is a part of Ben's everyday life. As his soccer coach and the athletic director at the high school who Ben interns for, he is Ben's role model who "calls Ben out on his teenage crap" and tells Ben to put his best into everything he does. As a family we decide that, rather than exploring a new part of the world, as we usually do on our vacations, we need to be still and return to a familiar place of beauty.

The return to Maui after so many years reinforces the continuity that coexists alongside the constant change. As the plane lands, we take in our favorite views. For me it is the hillsides on the slopes of the volcano. I know how to find them even from thousands of feet in the air. They are the same but much greener than the last time I sat in their lap. The windswept north shore beach, again, the same yet made different by the presence of many Hawaiian sea turtles, who I had not seen for many, many years. It is a dynamic landscape, always shifting as weather patterns and microclimates drift in and float out. Change is a part of beauty here.

We are again shaded by the afternoon clouds that always gather at about three thousand feet above Olinda in the late morning. I know these clouds. The high school I attended is located on an old estate named Manalei, "garland of clouds." Taking in the familiar views in their fullness allows me to focus in on narrower, immediate encounters like the noise of plumeria branches dancing as the wind moves them against each other, the gentle smell of their flowers wafting all around us. When we are above the clouds in the crater of the volcano Haleakala, "the house of the sun," we hike below the rim into utter silence and stillness. Up-tempo change falls on our skin when walking with dear old friends through pastures and native forests. Are we walking into and through clouds, or are they passing through us? Putting out food for lunch under the clouds gives way to eating it in the rain, dried by the sun ten minutes later. Ever rapidly shifting, we are inside what I receive as the "cloud sutra" that teaches impermanence to my senses.

We move through the clouds when my family and I fly above the native forest on zip lines. "I feel like a bird!" I shout to my family. It is glorious! We are alive-alive! I haven't been so happy or alive in quite some time. As I fly, I shout out loud the Amitabha mantra and Karmapa Khyenno! I pray that he is with me in this moment, enjoying all of this with his own deeper sensations. I have a moment here imagining I am one of his birds.

It fills me with joy I hope I can return to as an ever-present resource of care.

With all of my being, "I am alive! I am alive!" I am not fighting my cancer; I am living with cancer.

The four of us search for the brilliant red and yellow of native Hawaiian birds in a small forest glen. We walk through mist and then carry its drips with us on our bodies. Every day, stay inspired! Find ways to feel uplifted, joyful! These become my steps in living with my cancer.

I began my children's training in taking in beauty at a young age. When they were toddlers, I pointed out flowers, clouds, birds, hillsides, anything and everything that delights or soothes our senses. "Look at that, isn't it beautiful? It makes me feel like jumping up and down," I say to them as I point to a cloud made pink from the sunset on our drive home from soccer practice. When Ben was four and learning addition, he made up his own equations: "cloud plus rain equals rainbow," or "nest plus egg equals birds." Now they point out sunsets or other beauty sightings to me. Rebekah is a gifted photographer. Her keen, trained eye captures moments to be shared and remembered. There is so much beauty in this world, there must be more than suffering.

6. Grieving for and with Living Loved Ones

At the end of eighth grade, four months after my mom's death, I write a tepid poem around a metaphor of grief as a storm. It is my entry for a school literary contest. My English teacher's promise that anyone who won a contest prize could skip the final exam pushes me to overcome my fear and reluctance at revealing my vulnerability and sadness over my mother's death. The poem must genuinely express some truth of what I experience in the months following my mom's death, as I did win a prize, despite the unexceptional quality of the writing (the feedback comments said as much; I always remember criticism).

Likening grief to shifting patterns of wind and rain causing destruction or a gentle presence of barely noticeable mist, my poem forecasts that grief will change over time, weakening eventually, I hope, so that it is unnoticed. By that early age I have already lived in complicated relationships to different forms of grief: grieving for the dead; grieving for my assaulted, amputated childhood; and the ongoing presence of its trauma. With the perspective of time and aging I know that grief, like all things, is impermanent. I know that to some degree at fourteen too.

In my post-surgery reading diet, I ponder a sentence by the philosopher Paul Ricoeur in the notes for his final book, *Living Up to Death.* He wrote, as he was dying, "Grief is an emotion felt by the living; grieving the re/action of people pained by the separation from their dead loved ones."

With my diagnosis and prognosis, especially as it is intensified after my escalated diagnosis of grade IV glioblastoma in August 2017, Ricoeur's formula tells me I am, or will become, an object of grieving. Maybe my long career as a griever is coming to an end.

I don't often ponder sentences by French philosophers, but there is something about his formulation that pokes at me. As I repeat Ricoeur's sentence to myself on my walks with Biz, my thinking stumbles. I experiment with rewriting it to find a different movement, one more applicable to myself: "Grief is an emotion felt by the dying; grieving the re/action of those who are preparing for their death and are pained by the separation from their still living loved ones."

When I begin working on this book, I feel quite sure that I wouldn't focus on Buddhist narratives about grieving. I want to understand the perspectives illness can offer on impermanence as the mechanism moving the living toward death. But the boundaries between the perspectives of those who are grieving and the object of their grief are porous; I find myself moving between the two all the time. I don't grieve for myself. Well, not primarily. There are times when I mourn the loss of imagined future moments. It is not my own future, but the future of my beloveds who will no longer find me by their side.

There are many Buddhist narratives that push at a fixed boundary between the unchanging binary division between the living and the dead. Or, at least, they push against that barrier to such an extent that they create gaps for us to step through. The companions I meet in these stories help me to see a fluidity of grief that moves back and forth between the living and the dead; the past, present, and most importantly the future. Each prepares the other for how to live, how to die.

Stories about the deaths of the Buddha and of Maya, the Buddha's birth mother, are poignant, powerful examples of the fluidity of ongoing relationships between the living and the dead. Maya dies ten days after her son's birth. Stories in Sanskrit, Pali, and Chinese narrate their ongoing encounters throughout the Buddha's life, even after his death. Maya dies lying upon the side of her body her son emerged from. Eighty years later, the Buddha dies in the same posture.

To me, Maya's death most importantly teaches that relationships with loved ones form and reform, starting before birth and continuing after death. Maya's relationship with her son extends before and after the days she lives as his mother in this world.

Maya was the first being to whom the Buddha preaches the Abhidharma, the teachings that form the third pitaka, or corpus of his teaching. Following Maya's death she was reborn in Tushita Heaven; when the Buddha is ready to teach that third pitaka, he reunites with her by ascending to give these teachings to her, before traveling back to the human realm and repeating them to his monk Sariputa.

My experiences of pregnancy and giving birth offer their own unremarkable lessons of impermanence, suffering, and happiness in particular and deeply ordinary forms. While pregnant with Ben, genetic tests ordered by my OB (unbeknownst and unwanted by me) suggested a possibility that he could be born

with genetic mutations that would make his life short and painful. I clearly recall talking to him in my womb, in the aftermath
of this revelation, thinking it might be the only time we would
share together.

While walking to work on a perfect New England spring day,
I described to him all that delights me: crocus flowers making
their way through just-warming soil, budding trees, birdsongs,
crisp blue skies. I wished to infuse him with my joy and my
love. Ed and I sang to him together, "Me, you, and the chicka-
dees, holdovers from the wintertime." This one line is all I can
remember, but I still feel why it comforted me.

Those possibilities of disease turned out to be nothing. But
knowing every moment could bring either life or death per-
sisted. Each moment toward birth could and did also become
movements toward death. Life and love somehow become the
louder chords lifting us through our days.

The birthing experiences of both of my children's disentangling of our one body into two were dramatic ruptures. Neither
of my babies cried at birth; both of their skin colors were bad.
Rebekah's skin was so white and her lips so red that she resem-
bled a Japanese Noh performer; Ben's temperature was ele-
vated. Emergency codes were called, delivery rooms filled with
doctors whisking my newborns away from me. In those traumatic first moments of life I longed for them to be back inside
of my body where I could shield them from a world of suffering
and pain, back where we were one. Perhaps it was this jolt into
embodied separation that consistently reminds me up through
today that they are their own persons. My children constantly
change in their own ways just as our links to one another grow,
disconnect, and re-form.

Knowing the ever-present source of my death as something

that will never go away motivates me now to prepare them for my death and create the conditions for their flourishing after it. As I prepare for my death, I grieve for them. This is a flowing process changing year by year as they grow and their needs change. Recently, attending Ben's high school graduation is a triumphant celebration acknowledged in a hushed exchange between Ed and I during the ceremony. "I made it!" I whisper.

Ed encourages me, "You are here! Four more years, you'll be here at Rebekah's too!" Photos of our beaming faces capture the joy of living that moment together. I am here. This is the partial answer to our question of "When will I die?"

They need me. But the intensity of that need decreases at a rapid pace, and the form it takes changes too. When Ben is a young boy I come up with all kinds of strategies to help him work with his challenge with stress. I suggest visualizations to help him get to sleep. Together we create "Ben's Den" in his closet as a place of isolated retreat for stillness and much-needed alone time.

Now he develops his own strategies: working out at the gym, keeping a mini-garden in his room, spending time with supportive friends. I talk him through particular challenges when invited. Otherwise my job is to step back and let him grow. I am attentive, available, working to see him for who he is as he evolves. Each relationship grows at its own pace, as it should.

In a brilliant teaching on preparing for death, the Tibetan Buddhist teacher Mingyur Rinpoche identifies for us the first step: letting go of attachments to our loved ones.

I confide to a friend, "If it weren't for my kids, I'd be fine to die now." Is this true or bullshit? A way to soothe myself or an ego display for others? Have I prepared myself with Dharma practice? No. Prepared my husband for life without me? Not fully enough. Finished the scholarship to publish articles that might be of service to others? No. Finished this book, with the hopes of providing resources to others living with terminal illness or trauma? Not at this moment, but soon, I keep hoping.

Mourning for living loved ones is an effort to help them live into their future without me. It isn't determinative of course, but even a wish for vagaries of their future happiness, strength, courage, and equanimity, with a knowing heart that all will be possible without my presence, helps me lessen my attachment to the form of our relationship now, and I hope theirs too.

❧

I know I have to disentangle my attachment to my family as it is in its present form. Even before my (anticipated) death we are already evolving into new forms of relationships. I can pull my strings tighter or let go, living our relationships with the ongoing possibilities impermanence offers. As I often discuss with my college students, loving with nonattachment is not loving with detachment. Love is still present in our connections but lived with the fluidity of change.

An episode in the life story of the twelfth-century Tibetan Buddhist master Gampopa gives me ground to sit upon through this disentangling. While still a practicing physician—he would only later in life meet Milarepa and become his closest disciple—Gampopa was at one point away from home healing people struck by a plague. He returned to find his son and daughter mortally ill with the same disease. He carried the corpses of his children in his arms, one after the other, to their funerary place.

Imagine their bodies in his arms, their small arms, legs, and heads, falling limp toward the earth. Or maybe he held them tight, pressing their stilled bodies close to his chest. Imagine the intensity of his grief as he then tried, but failed, to keep his wife alive. She too was infected with the same disease.

As she died, his wife insisted that Gampopa vow not to remarry after her death. According to his biography, her wish for his future was so important to her that she would not let go of her life, despite the intense suffering in her body, until Gampopa agreed. This dying wish is easily misinterpreted. Just as a mother might not wish to be replaced by any other woman in the lives of her children, so too might a dying wife feel consoled by her husband swearing that she would always exist for him in that role, that she is irreplaceable.

Gampopa's wife's direction to him, however, can also be explored as a gift to him and his future. By forbidding him to remarry, she sets up the conditions for what he needed to do next. Gampopa's wife had seen a vision of his future that was the opposite of what their life together was. She tells him that his life as a householder must die with his family. Free of the burdens of dependents, he must leave the householder's life and become a monk.

Gampopa, true to his vow, took ordination and entered a monastery, becoming a highly learned scholar and a tremendously accomplished meditator. Only then did he hear the name of the man who would become his lama: Milarepa. The first moment Gampopa hears his teacher's name, his whole body reacted to the sound, directing him to seek out the great yogi. Once united with him, he received the entirety of Milarepa's teachings, which he then passed down to his own students—among whom was the First Karmapa, Dusum Khyenpa.

I imagine Gampopa's deceased wife as a shadowy presence in the time he spends with Milarepa, particularly in their parting, when Milarepa sees a vision of Gampopa as his lineage holder. As part of her dying, Gampopa's wife sent him in the right direction, into a future that his teacher, Milarepa, affirmed.

How had she known? Did she have a better insight into her husband's potential than he did? I imagine that could be true. Perhaps she was encouraging to him to follow a path that had already emerged as the right one for him. As she died, she grieved for the man who would outlive her. Her grieving was in service of him, not herself. She perceived a future for her husband that he might not have been able to see on his own. Maybe his sight was limited because he could not see beyond the patterns of his ordinary life. Maybe he would have remained near-sighted due to the haze of grief descending upon both of them.

In grieving for Gampopa in his life beyond her own, Gampopa's wife continued her relationship with him—and through him she continued her relationship to the Dharma. As I read it, Gampopa's activity was all made possible by his wife's dying care, by her active grieving for him.

With the weakest of parallels, I mourn for Ed's future. I want to care for Ed after my death. Unlike Gampopa's wife's wish that he not remarry, I hope that Ed will. When I first learned of my tumor, the summer before Ben's first birthday, I recommended to Ed particular women we knew as potential replacements for me as his partner and as a mother for Ben.

My help wasn't wanted. Not at all. He'd take care of his own romantic life as a widower, thanks very much. When I ask him directly, Ed responds, "The point, really, is that I don't want to plan for this." As the years have passed, and I'm still alive twenty-two years into our marriage, I've long restrained from verbalizing my recommendations, but it's still on my mind. I still find myself feeling let down when I learn that a woman I'd identified as an excellent fit was, in fact, already married.

Sometimes I find myself watching Ed sleep, and I'm overcome by sadness that he will be alone once I've died. I often find him hugging my pillow when he's gone to bed before me. He says he does that too when I am out of town.

"It's not a question of wanting to choose," he explained when I tell him of my silly second-wife mental database. "It's that you are irreplaceable."

I think I am replaceable. I might even want him to take a vow that he will remarry.

But I know what he means. Others may fill parts of life where I'd been, but connections are unique in their particularities. Our life together has formed as it has because we've made choices and reacted to unchosen intrusions—most dramatically, my cancer—the way we have. We hope for more; in some ways we have found it.

Ed has become my caretaker. He manages my appointments, my medicines, and tracks the questions and responses we've received over the many years of my cancer's transformation. At every consultation with our oncologist he prepares a sheet of paper for his note taking. At the top of the page he draws a happy face and a sad face with a box to check below them. The first few seconds after Dr. Lai's entry into the consult room is enough to check one or the other. Dr. Lai quickly learned to tell us what counts as good news—that the tumor is stable—immediately. The anxiety of learning what shows on the MRI scan is real and ferocious.

There are many stages of life interwoven with one another. Still to come: both kids moving out for college, giving us the time and space to focus on one another in the ways we did pre-kids.

But then it won't be a return; that doesn't exist anymore. We could never return to our energetic optimism that sprung from deep naivete in our early twenties. It would be a shift into yet another metamorphosis of our relationship, and it could take us away from each other rather than bring us together.

Ed dreams aloud to me of a retirement of spending months of every summer sailing off the coast of Maine, winters skiing. I get seasick, and I don't know how to ski. I dream of spending a bit of every season, save summer, at the transporting Jodo Shinshu Eikando Zenrinji Temple in Kyoto. He will join me there, perhaps spending his days looking for good Japanese stationary. I'll happily sit on the deck of a cottage, as long as it's screened, reading or maybe still writing. Peace, stillness, and the joy they offer. As I mourn for Ed, I hope that he steps into his future, knowing that whatever form it takes includes my love. My mourning for Ed is ordinary and humble. I want him to go on without me with my love and joy for the happiness that he finds there.

❦

In the Khmer Theravada tradition, Maya's death is described in Dharma songs with great depth of emotion. In one Khmer Dharma song that portrays her awareness that she will soon die, she sings a lament that she will be leaving her newborn child, Siddhartha, motherless. Without her, he will be lacking the conditions he will need as a newborn and those he will need later for his flourishing into adulthood. In this song Maya entrusts her son to her sister, asking her to care for him in her absence.

Her voice could be the voice of any dying parent, anticipating the needs of their orphaned children and doing what they can in their time before death to make sure those needs will be met after their death. In this song, it is an utterly selfless request. Maya asks to be replaced and trusts her sister to perform the tender acts of holding, bathing, and nursing her ten-day-old child. She confronts her imminent death as the reality of all impermanent things. Siddhartha's birth is paired with her death. She begs her sister, Prajapati, to always care for her newborn child: "Don't stop!"

These haunting lines of the Khmer lament, translated by Trent Walker, offers the dying, especially mothers and parents, an expression of their wishes for their living loved ones. Here Prajapati is referred to by the Pali form of her family name, Gotami.

> Nurse him and bathe his body
> Attend to him day and night
> Care for him like no other
> O my golden girl, don't stop!

This song feels so true to me in all its depth and complexity. While the acts she describes are the normal human care all babies need, her ability to focus on her child's needs and not her own loss is remarkable. Maya asks to be replaced as mother. From my own experience as a motherless child, Prajapati's taking her sister's place fills a gap—but only incompletely.

Fissures and cracks remain to remind us of the impermanence of even this most entwined relationship of mother and child. In Theravada stories, Prajapati is always named as his stepmother and aunt, never the Bodhisattva's or Buddha's mother. Every time Prajapati is qualified in these ways, Maya is a shadowy presence. While Prajapati's role as substitute mother remains until her death, it also shifts over time, sometimes in unexpected ways. She becomes the Buddha's disciple when he returns to his homeland as the Buddha and preaches the Dharma there. Later, after succeeding in convincing the Buddha to ordain her, Prajapati becomes an arhat—an awakened being—and the founder and leader of the nuns' Sangha.

Literary traditions hold that the deaths of the Buddha, his former wife Yashodhara, and finally his aunt Prajapati, all occurred within a short time span. As arhats, all three controlled the time of their passing.

Prajapati and Yashodhara both first inform their female disciples that they will soon die and instruct them that they should not cry. Their deaths are a part of reality, a universal experience of impermanence.

According to their cultural custom, Prajapati and Yashodhara first ask the Buddha for permission to die, and they ask forgiveness for any wrong they may have done. He gives his permission and his affirmation there is nothing to forgive. This points, in Prajapati's case, to her achievement in founding the nuns' order. Earlier in their lives, Prajapati had requested the Buddha's permission to allow women to go forth into monastic life. The Buddha had already described women as equally capable of attaining nirvana as men, but many in the community opposed the formation and argued that allowing women into the order would harm the Dharma. The Buddha repeats at this momentous occasion that the nuns are blameless, that there is nothing for him to forgive, not to assure these women but to right the wrong views of his monks.

Prior to his choice to die, the Buddha cares for his living loved ones by ensuring that still-present sexist views and practices are addressed at their deaths. Many interpret their choice to die before the Buddha as a sign of their emotional attachment to him; seeing his death would be too much for these women to witness.

"How foolish," the Buddha proclaims to anyone who doubts the strength and achievement of these women. The Buddha, of course, says it best as told in the *Gotami Apadana*: they passed away before him because *there are still* those fools who doubt that a woman can attain awakening. To root out that ignorant view he instructs both women to perform miracles before the crowds of monks and laypeople. In the Sinhalese tradition's telling of this episode, the Buddha also gives an account of his previous wife's attainment of all ten perfections that transform a bodhisattva into a buddha, before requesting that she perform miracles to cut down misogynistic ignorance. When Yashodhara performs her aerial miracles, taking different shapes in the sky, she shouts out triumphantly, "I am the nun Yashodhara!"

The Buddha declares that both Prajapati and Yashodhara are worthy of funerals at which a buddha will preside. He deems their parinirvanas—their deaths as fully awakened arhats—to be absolutely perfect, even more so than his own parinirvana will be, because a buddha will be present at both of theirs, while there will be no buddha at his own. The stories of these women's funerals describe him circumambulating their bodies and placing flowers on their funeral pyres. He marks them as objects of veneration.

Later, at the death of Buddha himself, his birth mother, Maya, who died after his birth, is present. News of his impending death had reached her in Tushita Heaven, and so she descends to the human realm to venerate her son. In Chinese versions of this story, Maya worships at his feet, upon which the Buddha sits up and gives a Dharma teaching on filial piety. It is a wonderfully mythic story, challenging me to learn from it that just because it wasn't "real" doesn't mean that it isn't "true." Mother and son, Buddha and Maya, are interconnected over the entirety of his life (and lifetimes before).

The longer I try to view my own impending death through the vantage point of these stories, the more I see that these familial attachments aren't real—or at least, they aren't the unchanging binds I thought they were. It's not attachment to my children I experience as much as it is my own dismay at being left on my own in my own childhood. That too isn't true. The loving generosity of many people, especially my friend Gerrianne, who finds and fills a role of second mother to me and is now "Nana" to Ben and Rebekah, filled the fissures created by my mother's absence. I wasn't formed by a single story. Yet I have long been clinging to a story of myself as the mother-orphaned girl, and I sometimes still struggle to throw it off.

To me, there is no way that feels right to fill in the holes that will be opened by my death other than to live fully now with my loved ones. I've read about dying parents who leave birthday cards or letters for their kids to open in the future. I instantly know I couldn't do that, although I respect people who confront their future absence head-on in this way. For me, in my efforts to die embracing my impermanence, I recognize that I don't know who my children will be in the future as they evolve and change. I mourn for my loss of this.

I miserably laugh at my own attempts at pretending I am catching a glimpse of what I'd see if I hadn't died. Ben posing for prom pictures with his girlfriend helps me imagine the caring, handsome partner he might become in the future to a woman he commits to as husband. Rebekah's bold reporting of sexual harassment at her middle school leads me to imagine a future of marching side by side as activists. They already are these things; we have already marched together, and with Ben, at a #Me Too march to end sexual harassment and assault. The conditions are there and already taking fruit. I see them, but they will change, make so many choices. What if my imagination of them now significantly misses the mark of who they will become? It might feel worse than the silence of my absence if my letters were written to people they never became.

Still, before my first brain surgery in 2002, I did something like that. I wrote a letter to Ben, who wasn't yet two. I wanted him to have something he could hold that recorded my thoughts just for him, written by my hand. I thought of it more as an object than a message. What can I possibly say other than "I love you, and I wish I were with you"? I didn't know who he'd be, what would bring our connection back to life.

My fantasy is that my children experience a unique form of love from me, a mothering, unconditional love. I've lived surrounded by these illusions. Maybe it's the romanticized standards of motherhood that suffocate women, stuffing them into a form of selflessness: being a good mother is supposed to mean a woman should sacrifice every dimension of her life and identity to mothering her child. A distinct memory of the delight and horror of this intermingling takes me back to the small bathroom in our rented Cambridge apartment, holding a year-old Ben.

"Who is this?" I asked, pointing to his chest.

"Mama!"

"No! Ben!"

"I am Mama."

"Who is this?" I ask again, pointing at him.

"Mama!" he said confidently. At that age he wasn't Ben without me. Could he be Ben without me at thirteen, when I had my first craniotomy? At sixteen, when I had my second? Yes, of course he could; I know that it would be deeply unhealthy if our identities were inseparable at those ages.

As is the natural, healthy process of impermanence, my son pulls further and further away from me as he grows up. Mothering with the knowledge that I was dying in a specific, known way, means for me to see my children's evolutions toward independence and adulthood as stages to be celebrated as nonattachment rather than the mourning of loss. My fierce desire to see my children into adulthood keeps me from mourning too much their movements away from childhood. Each progression into adulthood brings relief. I can be a part of gathering the conditions they'll need for their adult lives. As they begin to need me less and less, I feel the gravity of a premature death lessening too.

I mother with impermanence. Each experience is relished and then let go. And yet I'm waiting for the next phases of their lives to unfold so that I can witness them. I struggle with this form of desire. With me present or not, he'll be alright, she'll be alright, they'll be alright.

Still, being a motherless child is hard. It is still hard for me sometimes as an adult who is now eight years older than my mom was when she died. At times, even a sometimes-terrifying mother is better than no mother. Might it not be harder to be without a good and loving mother?

Here again, when I need to shift my perspective, my kalyan-amitra Damcho helps me do that. When I share this particular fear with her, she stops my flow of tears by teaching me to see that my love will always be with them; no matter how long I have been dead.

She says, "Your love is a condition of their being. It is not dependent on your presence. It is a source woven into their very being, it is not the only condition, but it will always be an important and present condition." This was her response, as I remember it. If not word-for-word accurate, it is very close to this: some things that people say to us we memorize the first, and only, time we hear it.

Love is a condition of well-being, of human formation and the capacity to live well with impermanence. I had idealized my love for my children as unconditional—meaning, to me, that it was based on nothing; it just was and always would be because they are who they are, nothing more. I learned to see my motherly love for my children anew: My love is conditional. It is already a condition of who they are; while that will evolve as all things must, impermanence doesn't mean that this condition of love will ever totally disappear.

The conditioned love of mother for child might be expressed as "With this, can be that." Having lived with this evolving love, then other things become possible. I hope these will include confidence, joy, selflessness, and so, so much more.

I wonder if my mother ever thought about what would happen to me and my sister if she wasn't there to care for us. It seems unlikely that she did; the statistics are that a majority of people don't have wills or guardians chosen for their minor children.

It is more than a clerical task. To write a will requires a willingness to acknowledge one's own impermanence, the reality that one's life leads inevitably to death. Then sign your name on the dotted line.

My mother was reckless with her life and the lives of her children too. In one of her rages, when I was three years old, she intentionally drove into a tree. Another time she dropped the garage door onto the hood of the car. And finally, fatefully, she caused the head-on collision that took her life and could easily have taken mine. Her future would likely have brought more jumps toward death or destruction. It is hard to imagine her planning thoughtfully for her death.

In my experience, mourning is not only a process like the progression of a storm (I'm saying to my thirteen-year-old self who wrote her award-winning poem on this theme). It's also a practice of attending to emotions, old or new, and bridging the distances between the mourner and the mourned. Mourning can give structure to a continuation and transformation of a relationship with our dead loved ones.

After my mother died, my father suggested we say the Jewish prayer for mourning every day for a year. We didn't make it the full year, as is the custom, but I recall a few of those moments as soothing, a time of caring for her even as her presence was quickly falling away. The even-toned reading of the mourner's prayer brought my father, my sister, and me together. It also covered over that horror of her final day, before the crash, when she ranted and screamed and I cowered to avoid her wrath, there in that very space we now said the prayer. This layering reminded all of us that there was much to mourn, and it was good for me to find my way to those feelings too.

Ed's mother, Cecilia, died four months after my diagnosis of grade IV cancer. Her voice was one of the first I heard after my surgery. I recovered so quickly I called our families together with Ed to give them our post-surgery update. In response to my simple "Hello, Cecilia," she screamed in delight, "Karen! It's you!" Then, getting my father-in-law's attention, "John! Karen's on the phone! Your voice sounds so good, I am so happy to hear your voice!" she told me, ending with, "I love you! I'm so happy!" before Ed took the phone.

In Ed's family customs, "I love you" is not as commonly said as it is in ours. She was a very loving woman, just not as demonstrative as I am. Hearing her delight that I was OK and that she loved me brought me joy in those immediate post-surgery days. These were the last words she said to me; it was the last time we spoke.

Her own health declined rapidly afterward. In the period that followed, when I'm flattened by radiation and chemotherapy treatment, the way she faced her own death inspires me.

In response to a diagnosis of a new form of cancer (she had survived breast cancer a decade or so before), she decided clearly and firmly against any further cancer treatment in her eighties. She gracefully let life go. She offered her loved ones the gift of clear instructions to protect them from future regrets or self-questioning. She wanted to die at home, and she did, lying under a blanket made by her mother. While I am still recovering, unable to leave home, Ed and our kids arrive at her home from across the country before she entered a coma. "You are here! I'm so proud of you!" she says to them. These are some of her last words. They got to hear her speak her love for them. Her pride in them is her encouragement she gives them as they live into their futures.

Ed, Ben, and Rebekah sit by her bedside in shifting combinations with Ed's brother, Chris, and cousin, Ceci, until her death. "Talk to her, she will hear your voices," the wonderful hospice nurse tells them. Rebekah, a great talker, keeps her company for a long time. As she lingers, the nurse encourages her family to leave for a while, explaining that many dying people will not die while their loved ones are present. "She may need your permission," she tells Cecilia's sons. My husband gives that to his mother before all of them leave the house for a short time. When they return a little later, she has left her body.

The ongoing chemotherapy and battering my body had just suffered factored into the heart-bruising decision for Ed and the kids not to make the long trip again to attend Cecilia's funeral. Damcho, who was visiting at the time, and I invite my husband and kids to join us in prayers to Amitabha, praying that he guides Cecilia in her first days of the process of rebirth, but they decline.

As much as they respect the sustenance I gain from the Karmapa and the lineage practices, they don't engage. In my experience, rituals remain just forms until faith, imagination, and belief transform them into the deepest form of trust. Without that, the Buddhist rituals don't work for Ed and our kids after his mom's death. Even with Damcho's assurances that preparatory training wasn't needed, they won't sit with us. At dinner, they give an unnecessary apology and explanation that they are glad that Damcho and I were performing those prayers for their beloved *abuela*.

Ed had a similar experience of ritual continuing the relational bonds between the living and dead when his aunt and godmother, Pura, died a few years earlier. He had been at her bedside too, together with her daughter, Ceci, his mom, and his brother, Chris, when her last breaths were taken. Her funeral mass was deeply meaningful to him. In that prediagnosis time, when I was still my former strong, energetic self, I flew from our home in California to New York with our then-young kids to join his family for the funeral.

Raised Catholic, Ed had not attended mass for a long time; yet the fluidity of movements and prayers rose out of him as we entered the church. He kneeled, making the sign of the cross before we sat in a pew. The priest conducting the mass had been a friend of Pura's. Before giving the Eucharist, he first spoke of the ways that Communion was taken not only at the altar but between friends over life-giving meals, such as those he had enjoyed at Pura's table many times.

Pura cooked meals sourced with items from all over New York City, visiting one neighborhood market for fish because she trusted that fishmonger, another for bread because it was a few cents cheaper; she would walk for blocks for the best peppers. When Ed went to the altar to take Communion during the funeral mass, our young son asked to go too. Ed took him, thinking he would just be observing, but when he reached out his hands to take the Eucharistic wafer, Ed put them down, whispering to the priest, "He hasn't had his First Communion," the ritual preparation for a Catholic to receive the host. The priest smiled at him and our son, bringing the spirit of Communion alive when he replied, "It's not important right now," and he placed the wafer in Ben's small hands. The form of the ritual is the container for the spirit or compassion it's filled with, a spirit of continuing love and connection.

At every church we visited a month later in Salzburg and Venice, my husband lit candles for his aunt and his mom ("I need prayers for me too," she reminded him). I love seeing him do these rituals in these beautiful spaces. They help me see his vulnerability and tenderness. I wasn't able to always see those beautiful qualities in him as I do now. Perhaps these rituals of mourning were the soil that fed these qualities. I feel so much gratitude for his tenderness in the present as he regularly draws upon this and other virtues as my primary caretaker now.

Just as I want to share with my family the ways I want to die and be memorialized, I want to talk together as a family about how they might grieve without the rituals of a shared religious tradition. I want to envision and leave our own rituals for the time following my death. Maybe we'll be able to imagine and create those practices together. Rebekah has begun to make this request to help her as she looks into a future when I am absent. We imagined making an interview video of questions she would want to talk about at different points in her life, or a photo album in which we record our memories.

I try to build the first steps throughout their lives, knowing that I was dying in a particular way for the entirety of their lives. One step has been our family communion around our dinner table; another, the awareness and sharing of beauty all around us; another, the expression of our love for one another expressed repeatedly every day. Every departure, every phone call ends with "I love you." I see the ways in which our expression of affection makes present our family connection and our shared commitment to it. This frequent repetition of affection does not weaken its affect. As the dying one in our family of four, it is a daily, simple practice of relationship. As I lay in bed waiting for sleep to come, I often hear Rebekah knock on Ben's door and say, "Goodnight, Ben. I love you," followed by his reply: "I love you too, Rebekah."

The dying gift a future to their still-living loved ones by encouraging them to take the first steps toward a future in which they are no longer present. At the deathbed the living give permission to the dying, "It is OK to go." This is permission from the mourner to the mourned. Reversing perspective, the dying—the mourned—create a future space for their loved ones by encouraging them, "It's OK to go on without me!" Go on into a future with my love and holding my confidence.

My Buddhist companions take me to this practice of mourning for my still-living loved ones by helping them find ways to mourn for me at my death. By building the courage to live with death, our relationships can take new forms as they move into a future shaped by trust and love.

"It's OK to go. It's OK to go on." This is the dialogue between the living and dying.

I hear this dialogue too in the medieval Japanese letters between a woman named Eshinni and her daughter, Kakushinni. The letters give us a glimpse into the life of an elderly woman and her daughter, as told from the perspective of the dying woman, who voices her own concerns and gives her assurances to her daughter. (We don't have the responses from Kakushinni).

Eshinni was the wife of Shinran, one of the founders of the Jodo Shinshu tradition in Japan. In a radical move, Shinran left his monastic life at Mount Hiei to rejoin the world of laypeople. Overturning the long history of celibate monastics, he married and became a father. Eshinni was both his wife and his disciple, and the letters, which date to after Shinran's death, are a continuation of Shinran's teaching on faith in the Buddha Amida.

Shinran taught that the ritual of reciting the name "Amida Butsu" is solely a means of expressing gratitude for one's inevitable rebirth in Amida's Pure Land. To be reborn there requires no practice at all; it is completely an act of Amida's compassion.

The letters from Eshinni to Kakushinni are written at a human level of communication between mother and daughter. They are full of the newsy kinds of tidbits we'd likely text about today, although the content is the details from a medieval life—her servant's daughter had gone to a different place; she'd received a robe her daughter had sent—and more serious issues of famine and death.

These letters challenge me as a reader. I lack the historical context, as well as expertise in the interpretations of Shinran's teachings on the nembutsu and faith. Still, as I read and re-read this collection of letters, I find I can't leave them. My imagination fills in what I don't know. Aware of that, I heed the call to be cautious and try to be explicitly aware that I am reading them in my own way with my own purpose. I make no claims about the significance or meaning of these letters beyond the way they speak to me as a mother preparing my own daughter for my death.

I imagine myself reading over Eshinni's shoulder, trying to see what she sees. Eshinni gives Kakushinni instructions in the mundane matters her death will bring—how she should manage the family assets—mostly servants—that Eshinni will leave behind. She also places her trust in her daughter to finish a monument she is building for herself and her husband. This is a mother's assurance of her confidence that her daughter will be well grounded in the world. The message, as I read it, is one of "Go on without me!" and "I'm proud of you; be confident in who you are; take my trust in you and carry it into your future."

She also works to steady her daughter in the personal but universal teachings founded by her father, Shinran. Continuing her husband's teachings, Eshinni prepares her daughter for life after Eshinni's own death by teaching her confidence in impermanence and faith in the awakened ones who receive the dying. She counsels that Kakushinni must stand firmly in her trust that her father was reborn in the Land of Bliss and live with devotion and gratitude to Amida Buddha for his grace of rebirth. Eshinni herself has total faith that she will join her husband in Amida's Pure Land. I imagine her deeply felt wish that her daughter could share her confidence, trust, and faith in her every moment. This, she says, will be the future we can step into.

As I read, I hear Eshinni speaking to me too: "Have confidence in the teachings you have received. Rather than questioning your faith, make the choice to be grateful for it." The Karmapa brought me to the Amida practice by instructing me to recite the Amitabha mantra. (Amitabha is the Tibetan form of Amida's name.) I felt he had met me at the Jodo Shinshu temple in Kyoto, as I describe earlier; my family all saw his face in a painting of Amida there. Ben and Rebekah had seen him there first. Maybe my confidence in the Karmapa's presence with me when I die isn't shared by my family, yet Eshinni tells me to step into it. It is a helpful reminder. I wonder if Ben or Rebekah will someday look at the photo of the Karmapa with his arms around them at our home in Redlands when they were young and remember his confidence in all of us

My beloved grandmother died when I was in graduate school.

Her decline happens slowly at first and then very quickly in her last days. My aunt Joan cares for her in her own home, with extraordinary love and respect. As signs of death come more rapidly, I travel from Cambridge to New York to visit. My dad comes from Maui to be with his mom and sister. I am there during Passover, shortly before her death. My happiest memory of the women in my family happens at that Passover. Arriving before the first seder meal, I try to help my aunt with the cooking. My aunt periodically asks her mother, who sat at the kitchen table, questions. "Ma, how long should I leave the matzoh balls in the broth? Ma, do you think the brisket should come out now?"

I know these are unnecessary questions; my aunt, herself a grown woman with adult children, has made these dishes over and over, year after year. Her questions lovingly make visible her dying mother's importance. She is our matriarch, our source of family knowledge and tradition. Her questions invite her mother to offer her blessing: "It's OK to go on without me."

At some point the three of us dance a hora, a traditional Yiddish dance, in small circles in the kitchen. There is a lot of smiling, a lot of kisses planted on cheeks. There is a lot of uncomplicated, pain-free love. What a gift.

As I prepare to leave the next day, I know this is our last time together, and that it is my time to say goodbye to my beloved grandma. We are alone together. She is lying in her bed, floating in and out of sleep. In a moment of clear consciousness, we hold each other's gaze.

She tells me, "I'm afraid."

I stroke her hand, kiss it. I kiss her check. "It is OK," I tell her, not knowing what else to say. Faith in something would have been so helpful in that moment. She is the first of her tightly knit sisters to die. It was always the three of them, so close, nearly identical in appearance and in life. As the eldest, she'd eventually be joined in death by the two remaining; of course, they would follow behind her. She probably would take little solace from that. As far I knew, she had no faith in what would happen next. Without words of our own, I quietly sing to her as she falls back asleep. A song comes into my head, "Joy Will Find a Way" by Bruce Cockburn. I know she's never heard it, but I know all the lyrics. Still, I didn't know its subtitle, "A Song about Dying," until later. I quietly sing to her: "Make me a bed of fond memories. Make me to lie down with a smile." I try to ease her fear by reflecting back to her the love she's given to me my entire life.

Her longing for living shifts, for me, into the love she gifts to me. Decades after her death, I carry it with me, always. I think of her almost every day; really, I do.

Her last moments of life were spent with her children at her bedside. My dad told me that soon before she dies, she looks at my dad and aunt and says, "Let's all give one last 'Oy!'"—a Yiddish expression of the everyday suffering of life. I hope joy did provide a way forward for her. Her love helps me shape a path that include steps up to joy.

Mourning for living loved ones is to give your care by imagining a future for them without you in it. It is to give permission, joy, and hope for an extended future, a future that will take its own course, but whatever it is, it will be imbued with joy and love.

7. Companionship
Follows Absence

While I participate in the trial for the experimental cancer drug in 2014, my days begin and end with a handful of pills that my husband sorts into a plastic box for each day of the week: morning, mid-day, and evening. Every two months I spend an hour chanting my mantras in the MRI machine at UCLA while it takes scans of my brain.

Then we meet with Dr. Lai, my neuro-oncologist. We talk over my seizures, wobbly balance, and ever-increasing levels of fatigue, and he considers modifications to my medications. I take these powerful pills because I trust his expert knowledge and commitment to his Hippocratic oath to do no harm. Dr. Lai selects them because he has confidence in the studies of their effectiveness. But some of this comes down to belief and faith. Am I having seizures? Seems like it, but likely of the smaller, short, break-through sort. And then if we get into questions about the cancer necessitating all these pills, there are more unknowns than knowns. I choose to continue to take these pills knowing how the side effects feel. There is nothing voluntary about having cancer.

The story of Buddha Sakyamuni's parinirvana, his final death in samsara, shifts from the universal patterns of involuntary birth, suffering, and death common to any living being to the unique aspects of voluntary death limited to extraordinary awakened beings: arhats, bodhisattvas, *pratyekabuddhas*, and buddhas.

Understandably, we might assume that the story of Gautama Buddha's death would have extraordinary elements, as did those of the arhats Prajapati and Yashodhara; remember, they flew through the air to display their realization before passing into nirvana. Yet while there are some of these elements, his death is mostly portrayed as humble and earthy.

The *Mahaparinibbanasutta*, the story of Buddha Shakyamuni's death in Pali narrative traditions, brings together the power of a buddha to shape an extraordinary death with the value of its seemingly ordinariness, including the final illness from which he dies. After decades of teaching the Dharma and leading the Sangha, Buddha Shakyamuni dies of dysentery from his final meal of spoiled food. It is an ugly death of intestinal pain, full of feces and vomit. Why encourage us to imagine these disgusting narrative details, which precede his final posture of lying peacefully on his right side with his head resting on his arms?

Here is a teaching on impermanence that pierces through all of our defenses that attempt to protect our living bodies. If the Buddha doesn't avoid the realities of impermanence, then how can an ordinary person? But still, a buddha dying from dysentery?

Why does this narrative demand its audience encounter this nuance? Here is a being who could die with any experience of death, and yet he voluntarily chooses this one?

To me, the Buddha's final illness is a story of companionship and of great compassion. Like us, in his human manifestation—

and unlike the beauty of his body in all other moments of his life—his body devolves. At the end of his life, his body becomes reminiscent of the old and sick bodies his father, King Suddhodana, had tried to hide from him on his journeys outside the palace. On seeing them he had asked his chariot driver, Chanda, if aging, illness, and death would happen to him too. "Yes," was the answer, and now he reaches that foretold moment.

The Buddha was cared for up to and after his death by his devoted, sweet attendant, Ananda (his name means "happiness" or "bliss"). For decades, Ananda was the person in this role taking care of the Buddha's physical and material needs. Ananda accompanies him everywhere, almost always by his side, hearing and remembering every teaching with attentive awareness.

When Ananda sees that the Buddha's death is approaching, he requests that the Buddha push it away and remain in the world. The Buddha's response to him is somewhat sharp. It was too late to ask that question. The Buddha had earlier given Ananda three opportunities to request that he, the Buddha, put off dying. Had he been asked, he could have delayed his death into a future so far away it might be described as infinite. But to do so he had to have been asked by a disciple at the proper time, and each of those three times Ananda had failed to take the hint that he might make such a request. There could not be a fourth opportunity, so now the Buddha will die. Ananda has been set up; in a way it's his fault that the Buddha died. That is quite a heavy load for Ananda to carry.

And yet how could it have been different? Ananda's failure to make the request makes way for an incomparable embodied teaching of impermanence. In the version of the story from the Pali canon, like all conditioned things, Buddha Shakyamuni is impermanent too. By his act of dying, the Buddha teaches this aspect of reality to its complete extent. Ananda carries the load of the Buddha's passing for all of our sakes. By not asking the Buddha to extend his life, Ananda makes it impossible for the Buddha to live on. While Ananda doesn't tell Buddha, "It is OK to go," by not asking him to remain, Ananda's silence has that effect. The Buddha can no longer chose his time of bodily death. That act becomes, to a degree, involuntary—like ours. This is a gift of generosity. Ananda models for us the moment we tell the dying, "It is OK to go," and the Buddha models the response, "It is OK to go on without me. You have the conditions to live in my absence."

The Buddha had taught Ananda how to care for him in his final illness years earlier through the care they had given together to the monk abandoned by his companions in their monastic hut. Now as old men, Ananda and other monks tend to the Buddha's dying body in the same way.

After bathing him in a river, Ananda sprinkles the Buddha's body with clean water and then, with greatest reverence, moves his hands over the Buddha's body to clean his skin. Next, he replaces the Buddha's soiled robe with a clean one and lays him down on his right side between two sala trees. This is his final resting place. As readers of these Buddhist stories, like in our own lives, we find ourselves returning to earlier moments for guidance in what to do now. The past prepares us for the present.

In Buddhist stories the Buddha's death leaves the biggest absence imaginable. Even though it is a necessary absence, it is mediated in different ways in different Buddhist traditions.

In the Theravada tradition, the Buddha instructs his monks and nuns that in his absence they will have the Dharma and one another; the laymen and laywomen will also turn to them, the monastic Sangha and to the Dharma that the Sangha will preserve. The Buddha's physical absence will be mediated by his relics, both bodily and material—his bowl, robe, and walking stick. Pilgrimage sites mapped onto the places of his significant activity will also provide geographic spaces to step into the memory of particular stories from his life's chapters. Pilgrimage, too, serves as a devotional tie linking past to present.

At his death the awakened members of the Sangha—the arhats, the people who have reached nirvana—are beyond grieving, but they are not beyond feelings of devotion for the Buddha. The great arhat, Mahakashyapa, had been away during the Buddha's death. Once he learns of it, he hurries to the funeral site together with a great number of monks. Laypeople charged with the funerary rites have already attempted to light the pyre upon which Buddha was lain, but no matter what they try, it will not catch fire. It is only once Mahakashyapa arrives and is able to venerate the Buddha's body that the pyre can be set alight.

The human and mythical speak side by side in the Buddha's death stories. One of the most touching of the humanistic stories again focuses on Ananda. After the cremation and dispersal of ashes, a weeping Ananda returns to the Buddha's *ghandakuti*, his "perfumed chamber," the Buddha's residence where Ananda had daily taken care of his physical and material needs.

Ananda once again performs all of his daily tasks as though still tending to the living Buddha: he makes the bed, prepares a seat, fetches water, and sweeps the hut. In allowing Ananda to care for him with these ordinary, everyday acts when he was alive, the Buddha had taught Ananda a method to grieve for him after his death. Veneration and grief mingled in a single act.

To perform such now-unnecessary acts of care after a

death—if they are mindfully performed—is a way of repurposing the everyday moments of care into ongoing bonds of presence. They become methods that the living can perform in their transformed relationship to a person now absented by death.

As described by scholar John Strong, Ananda's ongoing care of the Buddha's dwelling in fact did become the basis for a widespread devotional practice of sweeping the space before an image of Buddha and offering perfumed scents and flowers to create a ghandakuti for the Buddha in the devotee's own time and space. The absent Buddha becomes present and well attended to. Moving into this story and learning these actions from Ananda, a devotee in any time and space finds a way to be beside him as he serves Buddha.

As I hold these stories of Ananda close to me, reading and re-reading them, imagining the light, shadows, colors, scents, and movements, I feel lonely. I wonder, did Ananda feel lonely too? (I quickly caution myself, "Don't project your own emotions onto Ananda.") He does seem lonely to me, though. Sometimes particular feelings of loneliness arise in me that are connected, I think, to my cancer. As I attempt to comprehend the ways Ananda must disentangle himself from the Buddha, I see that I am tying my own threads to Ananda. It draws him closer to me as a companion and at the same time escalates my own feelings of loneliness.

This is one of the many times that I must pause as a reader and ask myself to be clear on where I stand in relation to the narratives. I am reassured that I am aware of the distinction between my place outside the story as an empathetic observer and the world inside Ananda's story. I can trace the ways that I bring my own experience into my reading. The Buddhist story is inspiring my own reflections on my experience, but not making claims about what I can know about Ananda's.

By reading and re-reading these stories in my hopes to see if there is a way to understand the loneliness I feel, a memory comes into focus, an episode that I haven't thought about in probably thirty years. It is an afternoon a couple of weeks after my mom's funeral. I let myself into our house and drop my bookbag on the kitchen floor. Hearing the thump, it brings me to the end of her funeral, when everyone shoveled a scoop of dirt followed by a lei—a flower garland so prevalent in Hawai'i—onto her coffin. Each scoop of dirt made a thump too.

It is 1982, so our phone was wall-mounted with a long curly cord. I look through the fridge for a snack while dialing the number for the office where my mom worked as a dental hygienist. "Hi, Laurie," I say to the receptionist. "It's Karen. Can my mom talk?"

I think about what I'm saying only as I say it. It's too late to retract the words. I want to cram them back into my mouth; shove them down my throat; let the acid in my stomach dissolve them.

"Oh, honey," Laurie says after a pause. Being addressed shakes me back into focus.

"I'm so sorry," I manage to croak out. "I wasn't thinking, Laurie, I'm so sorry." I hang up the phone as quick as I can; I cannot bear to hear her crying. The impact of this automated act was so powerful it entirely ruptures my illusions that the ordinary patterns of life apply in this time of painful, acute change.

Before my mom's death, I always checked in with her by phone after letting myself into our house and turning on the television to fill the silence in the house as I do my homework. Those were the bonds built by the seemingly insignificant acts of everyday life: "How was your day?" "What time will you be home?" Those were the automated acts and surface questions that make me feel cared for and connected.

Maybe I call my dad at his office instead, or maybe I just didn't have a post-school call anymore. I don't know what filled that gap of her absence. It was hard to grieve without something to do.

On another afternoon in that same time, soon after Mom's death, the phone rings. The voice responding to my "Hello?" says, "May I please speak to Roberta Derris?" My mom. Another cutting of the strings of attachment through the phone line.

"I'm sorry, she died a few weeks ago." Silence. This woman wishes she could take the words back into her mouth, cram them down her throat. "I'm so sorry," she says after a pause. "I knew your mom in Boston. I'm on Maui for my honeymoon. I wanted to say hello. She is such a great person. I'm really fond of her." My mom taught for a time at the Forsyth School of Dental Hygiene training dental hygienists. She loved teaching. This must be one of her students.

Now my family has our own patterns: My kids offer their foreheads or tops of their heads for a kiss with good nights. There is always a "Goodbye, have a good day," or "Hi, did you have a good day?" joined with "I love you." Many, many "I love yous" and many, many kisses on heads, on cheeks.

Ananda has to let go of his attachment to the Buddha, even as he continues to venerate him. If he cannot, he will not traverse the final steps to awakening. And until he does this, he cannot join the awakened monks planning to assemble for the first council after the Buddha's death. And they need him. Without him, the monks will be unable to recite the full collection of the Buddha's teachings. Ananda, as the Buddha's longest-serving attendant, heard more of those teachings than anyone else. Gifted with an extraordinary memory, his mind is the repository of the Dharma. But for his voice to be heard at the council, Ananda has to first attain awakening. Without his presence, the Dharma will not be preserved.

His brother encourages him onward with this worthwhile pressure. It is time to remove the final impediments to nirvana. In order to do so he needs to find solitude, to settle into existing without company. I can imagine him leaving the Buddha's dwelling place, sweeping away his footsteps as he goes through the door for the final time. He has to let go of the Buddha in order to join him and preserve his teaching. What a lovely paradox.

However, wherever he goes people seek him out. He is so companionable that people want to be near him. He is also a living link to the Buddha. But the greatest conduit he can give to the most people for the greatest expanse of time is to recite the Buddha's teachings, sermons that will form the *suttapitaka*, the corpus of the Buddha's teachings (containing many of the stories I've retold). Responding well to a deadline, as many of us do (I know I do), in solitude he attains awakening. Now an arhat, he can recite the sutras at the first council.

Every time we hear or read *"evam me sutam"*—"Thus have I heard"—at the beginning of a Buddhist sutra, the "I" is Ananda. Every time we form these words with our mouths or receive them with our ears, Ananda is with us, communicating the immediacy of hearing the Dharma from the Buddha for the sake of us all.

Ananda must overcome his attachment to the Buddha so that we can have Buddha's Dharma and Sangha. Before the Buddha dies, he sets out these two jewels as that which will fill the gap left in his absence. There is no way to capture the diverse ways in which Buddhists have lived with the Dharma and Sangha in the Buddha's absence. The mediation through them of the Buddha's absences gives rise to more texts and to rituals of devotion.

Like the Buddha, the other two jewels of Buddha Shakyamuni's *sasana*—that period in which his teachings will abide—the Sangha and the Dharma are also impermanent. Cosmological texts tell us that eventually they too cease to exist. That period, which we can only imagine, might seem to be the loneliest time of all—when the world is without any refuge. Buddha Shakyamuni's sasana is gone, but another will arise when the next buddha, Maitreya, is born in the world. The space between buddhas is a tremendous, empty gap when none of the three jewels are present—no Buddha, no Dharma, no Sangha. Yet the freedom and dynamic creativity of impermanence brings other forms of presence into those empty, empty times.

◈

Pratyekabuddhas are yet another category of awakened beings that Buddhist stories invite us to meet. They offer a beautiful model of companionship, one that only comes into our world when it is absent a buddha's sasana. These are awakened beings who attain liberation without the aid of buddhas—which explains why they are not arhats. References to pratyekabuddhas are found in Mahayana sutras, where they are usually derided as deeply inferior to buddhas and bodhisattvas because they are viewed as lacking the compassion of these other two types of awakened beings. They have a more important presence in Theravada traditions, especially in Pali commentary. I am fascinated by their companionship with one another. Unlike the highest form of budddha (*samyaksambuddhas*), who can never coexist with another buddha, pratyekabuddhas are often told to be in companionship with one another. They are also present for us in times when the three refuges are absent. When discussed in Buddhist studies scholarship they are, in my opinion, misinterpreted as "silent buddhas" who are isolated and withdrawn from others..

Based on the stories from the Theravada tradition, where they are known as *paccekabuddhas*, they care for us when there are no refuges in the world. The stories of paccekabuddhas help me imagine a beautiful model of companionship in a time of absence, a time when there seems to be no refuge to turn to. They are so appealing to me now as I fear leaving my loved ones. They represent to me the possibility of easing loneliness and finding companionship when I feel alone and afraid of my monstrous brain cancer.

One of my favorite stories of this sort is about a king of Benares whose awakening as a pratyekabuddha is the result of the intervention of four other pratyekabuddhas. They had shared a previous lifetime together as five pratyekabuddha-bodhisattvas—proto-pratyekabuddhas—during which they made identical aspirations to attain a pratyekabuddha awakening together. The awakening of a paccekabuddha will be less spectacular than that of a samyaksambuddha (a full and perfect buddha) and their *pratyekabodhi* (their realization) will also be less than a buddha's, but together they will bridge the void created by the total disappearance of Buddha Shakyamuni's sasana.

The relationship between this small community of pratyekabuddhas thus extends across lifetimes. In the story we learn that in their present form, four of the five are dwelling together on the slope of Mount Gandhamadana, the home of all pratyekabuddhas, a space set apart from our world but reachable for those with the requisite spiritual powers to journey there.

One day, as they are enjoying the *brahmaviharas*—the sublime mental states of kindness, compassion, sympathy, and equanimity—the four pratyekabuddhas realize their fifth companion from their previous lifetime has yet to attain awakening. Also, they see that their companion is facing significant obstacles to awakening. He is in desperate need of their help.

From their remote residence in Gandhamadana, the pratyekabuddhas' supernatural vision enables them to see that their companion has been reborn as the king of Benares. He is a fearful king. He sees danger all around him. At night, he runs through his palace, terrified of the sources of harm that he dreams are surrounding him. He points his sword at invisible enemies who he believes are intent on killing him. His court ministers suggest that the way to defeat these imagined threats is to offer a tremendous animal sacrifice. It is at this crucial moment that his companions from their shared previous lifetime leave their home on Gandhamadana and fly down into our world and enter Benares.

Then the pratyekabuddhas having seen the assemblage of thousands of animals soon to be ritually slaughtered, realize: "If he kills these animals and is coupled with the resulting karma, it will be difficult to teach him the truth of enlightenment. Come along then! Let's cautiously go to him so we can make him see."

Once in Benares, the four pratyekabuddhas walk through the city begging for alms in the appearance of mendicants—holy beggars. Because the world is absent a buddha and his Dharma, there is no Sangha, and thus there are no daily alms rounds of monks and nuns to provide a field of merit for laypeople. For the pratyekabuddhas, this alms-gathering is instrumental for their specific goal of teaching the Dharma, specifically the four brahmaviharas, to the king of Benares in order to awaken him to the enlightenment of a pratyekabuddha.

When the king first sees the mendicants from his palace balcony, he instantly feels love for them and sends his attendant to invite them to his palace. Once he gives alms to them, the king asks, "Who are you?"

"O great king, we are called 'those of the four directions.'"

"O venerable sirs, what does this mean, 'those of the four directions'?"

"O great king, there is no fear or terror for us anywhere in the four directions."

"O venerable sirs, why don't you have fear?"

"O great king, by cultivating loving kindness; by cultivating compassion; by cultivating sympathy; by cultivating equanimity. Because of this we aren't fearful."

The pratyekabuddhas then teach the king how to be one who is truly free of fear through the practice of the brahmaviharas and thereby bring the king to awakening.

One of his courtiers then enters the hall and addresses their king in normal fashion as "king." He replies, "I am not a king," prompting the confused man to ask, "Who are you, if not the king?"

The king replies that he is a pratyekabuddha, a person free of fear in the four directions. Passing his hand above his head, the king is bodily transformed, instantly having the appearance of a pratyekabuddha with shaven head, robes, and the requisite objects allowed to a renunciant. It is as if the king sheds an outer identity to reveal his true, inner form.

With all five companions in shared forms as pratyekabuddhas, they fly back to their collective home on Mount Gandhamadana.

There is a mural in the monastic hall of Wat Suthat, a royal temple in the center of Bangkok, that depicts this story as told in the commentary to the *Dhammapada*. It is painted with beautiful detail, including a scene of the king pointing his sword at his dream enemies. My favorite scene in this very unusual mural is the rendering of these five pratyekabuddhas in flight as they voluntarily leave this world for their collective dwelling place on Gandhamadana. The former king is last in the aerial formation. The fourth looks over his shoulder, as if he is checking on and encouraging his new companion during the journey to his new home. The companions ensure he is guided to where he needs to be.

Gandhamadana is a place of peace and beauty. There are caves for solitary or group meditation, lakes, and a monastic hall (depicted as the one where the mural is painted) where everyone gathers whenever a new pratyekabuddha arrives. When these five companions land, they enter this hall and take their seats, arranged by seniority. When invited, this newest pratyekabuddha recites his awakening verse to the others.

On their own, or with small groups of their companions, pratyekabuddhas dwell in the brahmaviharas. Animals, including elephants, act as their attendants, just as the elephant Parileyaka attended the Buddha when he left the quarrelling Sangha. Particular kinds of winds clean the ground, making it perfectly smooth, and blow away the flowers that fall as offerings of beauty and scent, just as Ananda and the devotees in the Sangha performed the ritual acts of cleaning the Buddha's ghandakuti.

Gandhamadana is also the place that pratyekabuddhas return to in order to take their parinirvana when a bodhisattva is born into the world for his final lifetime, in preparation to become a full and complete buddha. Since pratyekabuddhas can only exist when there is no buddha, the final birth of a bodhisattva in the world must signal their exit from it. With the conditions for a new sasana in the world, the pratyekabuddhas know that their bridging role is complete. It is no longer a time of absence. The conditions for fullness are present once again. Those pratyeka-buddhas alive in the world at the time of the bodhisattva's birth gather on Gandhamadana. They might spontaneously combust, or they might jump off a cliff, where their bones will remain as relics falling upon the bones of previous pratyekabuddhas of past eons.

Across gaps of time and space there are those who care for us and each other. The universe is even more generous, compassionate, and responsive than we can imagine on our own. Through my practice of reading, I remind myself of this.

❦

In attempts to investigate and ameliorate my loneliness, I join some online communities of people also living with glioblastoma. I am daunted by the courage I have to find in order to reach out to people with whom I share an embodied experience. But these are people I have never met directly, nor am I likely to. I write into a Twitter feed, something that's new to me and facilitated by my kids.

"How does loneliness feel different with cancer?" I ask. Suzanne writes back, "I'm so sorry you have to ask this question. Loneliness feels even more devastating with cancer." Another person responds to my disappointment that people aren't seeing me when they say I look good: "Why do you expect them to see you?" It is a good, pointed question. What are my expectations of companionship that would make me feel less alone, less devastated?

I'm scared to join these sessions. What if I feel even more alone afterward? But I don't; the presence of a longing for community and companionship is easily felt though shared experience. Still, just because we have the same disease doesn't mean there isn't a lot of difference among us. When a question is raised on how the disease is affecting family relationships, a few of us talk about children, but a few don't have kids, and for those of us who do there's a big range of children's ages. The moderator skillfully bridges the differing particulars so that we can see each other's situations.

I feel lonely sometimes because I assume people who love me can't understand what I'm going through because (thankfully!!) they don't have my form of cancer. I need to embrace their companionship across this difference. Of course, I must. This has been a strange emotional maze, but I've spent a great deal of my academic career trusting that we can learn across difference.

Loneliness is not lacking the companionship of people who occupy the same cancer experience as I am living with. Loneliness for me is dreading feeling alone. My dear friend Sarah, a skilled psychotherapist, shares her perspective with me that loneliness is being without an internal companion. Her definition connects instantly to a teaching by the Karmapa: When you need a friend, acquaint yourself with your own positive qualities.

Knowing oneself over time, through attentiveness to the present as well as reflecting on the past, is an antidote to loneliness. We are always companions to ourselves. My work is to make myself a good companion. After my most recent diagnosis I give myself a talking-to: no melodramatics; no feeling sorry for yourself. Revision: notice the suffering of others; if you still feel sorry for yourself, well OK then, but keep revising.

This is finding companionship through a challenging process. Yes, I started out thinking that I would only find companionship with those who had an embodied experience like me, thinking that no one could understand what it is to feel continuous illness unless they wake up every morning feeling uncomfortable, exhausted, and off balance. "No!" I shout at myself. "You are wrong!" There is so much generosity around me; I must be open to those offerings. There are many forms of companionship as experiences of life constantly change. The plentiful forms of generosity introduce me to my virtues as well as bringing my faults into my field of vision. Being a companion to myself requires both affirmation and regret; a full consciousness keeps me company.

A few examples: A friend of a friend hosts me in his San Francisco home before and after my third brain surgery in August of 2017. He gifts me a beautiful and comfortable place to prepare for and recover from my surgery. There is no reason to do this for me other than that he can. The world is even more generous than I imagine—or work hard enough to see. My best friend, Kelly, takes care of my kids during my second and third surgeries. What a difficult act of care I request of her. I didn't hesitate to ask; she didn't hesitate in saying yes.

I am in awe of the imaginative ways she transforms my then-ten-year-old daughter's anxiety while I'm in the hospital into an act of fun by asking her to make a public-service-announcement-style film on what you don't do when your mom is coming home from the hospital after brain surgery.

They make a hilarious film on her phone that lets Rebekah

express and feel all of her fear while laughing uproariously. My cute girl looks straight at the camera. "When your mom just had brain surgery, you don't ask her if she wants her hair done! You don't throw a dance party for her arrival. You don't jump on her bed." And so on. How brilliant to generalize the situation. The movie lets Rebekah know that she's not alone in having a sick parent. Other children also have to modify their behavior around their sick parents, and her advice film could help them too. I reflect back on Kelly's brilliant care for my daughter with so much gratitude.

Companions show up in so many forms. After my second surgery, Charlie sent me books, lots of books. Delivered onto my front porch several times a week. It came to me that this was his form of being a Jewish mother who tells her sick child or friend "*Es, es,*"—"eat, eat." Charlie's gifts of books said to me, "Read, read."

And I did: novels, poetry, the work of naturalists, some memoirs. Each book he picked out for me, maybe something he was also reading, was so that we could talk about it when I had enough energy. The world is more generous than I had known. Each author he introduced me to becomes a new companion. Each time I'm reading, Charlie is present with me, as he will be when we talk about the book. His generosity also appears in the absence of expectation that he'll benefit from these conversations. I fear I can't keep up with his brilliant observations and arguments. But he never signals that. I'm the only one comparing. And yet I imagine he is fearful of losing me, one of his companions, to this disease too.

I sometimes forget my diagnosis and prognosis. Forget? Not quite. It's more like they are not bearing down on me like a boulder carried by a landslide. There is breathing room to imagine myself in the future as an old woman; time feels more spacious then when I have less to do, fewer responsibilities. But who knows, maybe I have more. My past feels longer.

When I slip into this kind of reverie of the future, I know I must return to my reality. The smallest thing can bring me back into my embodied present: the icy sensation in my veins, a sensation I sometimes get from my neuropathic damage; hearing a story about a colleague's friend who was doing well with her treatment and then suddenly died; reading an op-ed in the *New York Times* by a woman living with cancer who shouts through her printed words: "Don't tell me I look good! I feel horrible." My reaction: "Yes! Truth, sister!" Those voices, signs, etc., are all *dakini* voices, delivering their messages to me while pointing at the present: I hear their voices telling me, "Don't avoid the knowledge of your truth. And more, trust in the opportunity to return to impermanence."

I begin to resettle into my cancerous body right then. I regain my confidence to confront fear and discomfort. I also check my calibration to go on oriented by love rather than fear.

Bizarrely, I look back on the seven weeks of concurrent radiation and chemotherapy with some longing. It hurt, but each day became stripped down, focused on the few essential things I simply had to do. I woke up, got to the radiation session. I walked the dog, if I was able, took my medications, and got a little food down. Getting through the radiation, going for a walk, eating, then spending time with my family and friends—and that was it. That was a day.

The radiation treatment and the pain that followed it deepened my practice; silently reciting my mantra and following my breath was my best approach to managing my fear and discomfort. Just lie still. I had to lie still during the radiation treatment. I lie still in my bed in the hours that followed. Move breath to every part of the body. Does my breath reach my toes, my fingertips? The top of my head? Do I feel it in the left foot and arm where pain lives? Yes. Good. Sensation still present. All I need to do is be still. I can do that.

During that fall I hear birds singing all around me. I hear so many birds of great variety visiting our neighborhood, as they likely had before, unrecognized by me. I hadn't heard their voices together before. The music had been there, as am I, absent a listener. Now, their music soothes me, inspires me. Accompanies me on walks or when I lie still. The birds singing the Dharma in Amitabha's Pure Land will be even more beautiful than this.

Other forms of companionship arise from my senses and consciousness. My dreams give me the longed-for presence of my lama. I haven't been able to see him for over two years. I note the intensity of my wish to see him. I try to shift to feeling gratitude for the extraordinary experience of spending so much time with him in this lifetime. It is a gift of immediate presence that few receive. Gratitude and contentment are my current focal points. I feel deeply a growing confidence, trust, and devotion when Karmapa appears in my dreams.

Some parts of the dream are recurrent and very simple: he is present, I see him in a space, usually a space I do not recognize. But I see him clearly. Another aspect of the dream: I am not successful in being physically in the same space as him. I didn't show up in the right place at the right time. But I see him clearly. I describe this as a transcendent perception of reality—a view beyond the material or "rational" opens my experiences to the "really real." This is the Reality I can experience when I free my imagination from analytic thought for a time.

Most extraordinarily, shortly before my second craniotomy (and third surgery), His Holiness calls me. Thankfully, I'm prepared when I answer my phone and hear his voice; his close assistant had just emailed me for my phone number. He has a small, simple task of writing a short letter he asks me to do. I told him my surgery would be the following week. He acknowledges that. I ask him to pray for me. "Of course, always." There was no need to ask. It is a lesson to stand upon my confidence, trust, devotion.

The next day I complete the small task I had been given. Many people felt confused about why I was being asked to do anything with my surgery coming up. It was perfectly clear to me: This ask was a gift of great compassion that made me feel connected to my lama, enabled me to serve him and earn merit right before my surgery.

About a month later, I receive another short phone call from the Karmapa. First, he makes a statement: "The surgery went well." It is decidedly not a question. Responding, I say, "Yes. The surgery did go well. As you had told me, my fear of it was much worse than the experience. I start radiation and chemotherapy next week." He acknowledges that information with something like "ah" or "yes." It felt to me that the news of the next step of treatment and its timing is an affirmation of something already known. It is an extraordinary love to know my lama sees me as I go through each part of my treatment. I also receive a second invitation to do a small project that will only take a half-hour or so. Again, it is a joyful focus as I prepare for my next phase of treatment. I feel gratitude to be of service. It is the perfect orientation for each day into my future.

After the intense seven-week treatment I stumble through daily life, going back to teaching and chairing my department and the routines of a full life. Some days feel impossible; stumbling feels more like crawling. When a new source of stress is added, breathing, while physically still possible, feels impossible. Noticing this, I take a deep breath, I breathe.

After an unusually tortuous day, during which I fail to prevent a difficult confrontation with a colleague, I wake up at 4:30 a.m. with my mind in knots. In the few hours of sleep that follow, I'm inside a vivid dream of being somewhere with the Karmapa. He gestures permission to approach him. Standing before him feels as if he encircles me with his arms. I sob as my bowed head both falls and is held aloft. I am protected by him as the toxins of anger, enmity, and ill will drain from my body with my tears. When I wake up, I feel that I am in the presence of my lama. With that strength of the dream-like experience I can reorient myself from fear toward love.

In the three years now since my diagnosis of glioblastoma, every bimonthly brain scan shows the cancer is stable—no growth, no new tumors. As we say goodbye to Dr. Lai, who is as openly delighted as we are, I send out the results to my considerable circle of loved ones. "Good news! The cancer is stable!" This is our good news; given the limited treatments that exist now, we do not anticipate being able to hear, "There is no sign of disease. You are cured; the cancer is gone."

I tell my three closest friends about my dreams of the Karmapa; even though they are avowed atheists, through their love for me they can move into an imaginative space to see my dreams as I do. Each of them cries a bit, grateful that I have this resource of care to help me, to help all of us.

I dream again of the Karmapa. When I see him, somehow, I know he was in such a deep state of mindfulness that he could merge his consciousness with every living being; he perceives what they perceive. Then, in my dream I could see from his perception a great bird (maybe a vulture or eagle). Gliding on wind currents, circling high in the air, above craggy mountains and high steep valleys. After this dream, I am at ease: he must know what I am feeling, my activities. Faith empowers confidence that all I need to tell him is already being communicated. He knows through his ability to merge his consciousness with all things. He tells me through the gifts of dreams. I experienced this as a transformation of the canonical form. It moves from "Thus have I heard" to "Thus have I imagined." I wake from my dream both aware that it is a dream and also feeling my embodied experience: Freedom, beauty, companionship!

8. *"Not Dead Yet"*

"**N**ot dead yet." It's a quip from a Monty Python skit that Ed and I repeated frequently with naive humor in our early twenties. We sometimes say it now as a sarcastic declaration leading to our genuine focal point: "Still living." It's become our springboard for reflecting on gratitude, awareness of the present moment, and living into the future with determination and purpose.

Damcho told me a story long ago, which she had heard at Sera Monastery in southern India. A lama there, Geshe Lopsang Donyo, would walk up behind people and say, "You die today? OK? You ready?"

I remember this story for its outrageousness, the penetration of the question, and my wondering about the persons who could affirm that yes, they are ready today. I want to say yes. It's a lie for me to say yes. But the question prompts me to ask my own questions: What is the scope of death today? What is the form of the death taking place within that scope?

In Damcho's story I know that it's a question meant for me, even though it wasn't directed particularly at me. As with every story, observed as it is spoken, written, or experienced through the filters of place and time, it is meant for us if we let it be alive to us.

This story jumped into my mind just last week when my husband, daughter, and I help Ben settle into his new life at Connecticut College.

Saying goodbye to him is much harder than I thought it would be. After setting up his dorm room, at the very end of a long, hot, and humid day of menial tasks, it gets close to the time for us to leave. The orientation schedule for parents was wonderfully clear about this: "Six p.m.: parents depart." I am distracted at the college president's reception. I want to give her my approval of her address on the college's mission of a "Liberal Arts Education in Action." I waste precious time as I stand in the crowd afterward trying to catch her eye.

Ben repeatedly grabs my elbow. "Mom. This doesn't matter. Can we please spend this time together?" Regrettably, he has to ask me a few times. Finally, I see what I'm doing and not doing and follow him as he takes us for a walk to a quieter section of the campus green. A breeze comes up, cooling the air; the light softens to a golden hue. We give him our final, funny words of advice, hoping to reduce the intense emotions we all exude. Many, many hugs. After a family circular embrace, one of us, I don't remember who or what precise words they used, brings the depth of our family love into our circle by launching one of our family rituals: we put all of our pinkies together and then call out "zip" as we raise our hands into the air. We'd been doing that for years since the kids were toddlers. Our family was zipped together and now is zipping apart, I guess. At this moment, though, there was no interpretation of our ritual, just spontaneous action and love. My tears flow, as do Ben's. I watch him walk away from us into the campus where he will meet a group of students in a few minutes for his next orientation event. He looks so alone to me—but he's not. He is surrounded by a cinematic golden light. I stand watching him until he passes over a small incline in the path and he's no longer visible to me.

"You die today. OK? You ready?" I experience the death of my daily mothering to this incredibly lovely son. A death of a part of me as an ever-present source of support for this being. "Let go! Let go!" I say to myself. Disentwine your attachment to your son. Those binds are dying as new strands are forming. "OK?" I will be. I am.

"Victory!" my husband declares. "We have given him what he needs to be in the world and be a part of it. Victory! You are here to be a part of it!" All true!

As one thing dies it becomes compost for something else to grow. My illness and the side effects of the medicines I take separate me from my kids on our family adventure in the Azores, directly preceding the college separation. Exploring volcanic caves, crater lakes, walking to thermally warmed ocean pools are all too physically challenging for me now. I encourage them to go on without me. I sit on the side of the forest trail listening to birdsongs rather than truncate their hike to the crater lake a few miles down the trail. Each of these days and sat-out experiences is a little death from my cancer in the frame of my future death.

My attempts at composing poetry have been few and far between. How few have I written since that middle-school poem on the storm of death? I love poetic form and rhythms, the attention a poem can draw to each word and its placement. I am the admirer not the composer. Sometimes, though, I have an experience that inspires a mostly formed poem. If I have the energy to write down what I hear in my mind, I capture an experience in what feels like a foreign tongue signaling, to me, the uniqueness of what I've seen, heard, and felt. I am content with the few amateur poems my experience demands.

Yellow Finches (written during my recovery from my second craniotomy in fall 2017)

> The Ash tree outside my kitchen is full of yellow
>   finches this morning.
> Flashes flitting
> Between branches
> Drinking last night's raindrops from green cups.
> Crumpled autumn leaves finally fall.
>
> Call them Ben or Rebekah,
> Rebekah or Ben.
> Let them fly together
> In warming sun.
>
> Find your strength as I found mine.
> Write your own story.
> Death and grief
> Need not be
> Central themes

This family time on a beautiful island in the Atlantic is an unexpected lesson in contentment. Walking down through this beautiful forest as a family is the stuff of my dreams. The stillness and quiet of sitting in the forest listening to the birdsongs invites reverie of its own, as it encompasses watching my loved ones' return up the switchbacks, waving from below. Let go of the ever-present desire for more; be content. It's a new and challenging practice. I can't will my formerly strong, well-balanced body back; I've tried, too many times. Confronting loss, frustration, giving in, letting go, finding my new limitations. The bruises all over my legs give visible evidence of the cost of pushing against those new limitations.

The only hope I bring to this place is swimming with dolphins in the wild Atlantic. A boat will take us to where we might encounter dolphins. If the dolphins swim toward the boat, we can then slip into the water and swim with them.

Some distance from shore there are hundreds of dolphins. People on the boat slide down the pontoons and swim among them. I've been snorkeling most of my life; I'm a strong ocean swimmer. I descend into the water and all that seems to be gone. Floundering, I'm taking water in through the snorkel. Raising my head above the surface to gasp for air, my mask loosens and my eyes sting from the salty water. Climbing the few steps of the ladder back up into the boat, I fall backward, slamming into the water. I can't do it. Everyone else excitedly describes what they see under the water. I see nothing. Time and time again I can't put the necessary actions together. I am so frustrated. Growing up on Maui, former me was a strong ocean swimmer and experienced snorkeler. One of the boat staff goes into the water with me, guiding me, taking my hand. But this time I take water into my lungs, twice. It feels like I might drown. As I swim back to the boat, I panic. My focus shifts from seeing dolphins to staying calm and breathing through the snorkel. I get back into the boat panting for air.

One last try. I encourage myself: stay relaxed, go easy. Before I begin searching for the dolphins, I hear them. Keeping my body in that spot, I let go of movement and sight and stay still, listening to the clicks of their language. There are so many voices. I hear them all around me calling. Responding? Greeting? Or calling farewell? Voices all around me that I cannot see, and I cannot know. I feel encompassed by their voices. Finding my own stillness, I am encircled with songs of companionship.

Hearing the voices, so many voices, hearing but not seeing, far away and yet right there. It is something like bringing Maya, Prajapati, Eshinni, Ananda, and the Karmapa into my presence right now.

It is beautiful. I feel delight. A few moments later a large pod of dolphins approaches, swimming in circles around the boat. Kneeling down at the side I watch them ascend and descend in rapid simultaneous movements. I see the spots on their silky, skin; the varying colors of their bodies and fins. Some ascend into dazzling jumps. They seem to play with great delight.

Back on shore, we four compare experiences. Ben and Rebekah's is the one I hope to remember best: The two of them are swimming together a distance from the boat when they see a pod of twenty to thirty dolphins swimming in a circular pattern as they descend deeper and deeper, moving ever deeper into the remarkably blue ocean.

I know in the future I will recount this memory to them, even though it didn't happen to me. I am moving into their experience now by asking them to describe it to me multiple times. "How far above them were you? How many dolphins formed the pod? They followed each other in a circle as they swam deeper? Were you close to each other? What did it feel like?" Maybe these questions will help them remember it. To me, their amazing shared experience marks the beginning of their adult friendship.

"It's much more impressive seeing them above water rather than below, Mom," Ben says, compassionately trying to console me. I describe hearing the sound of their voices. "It's OK. I'm content. I really am." At first my words attempt to convince both of us, yet as I reflect on my experience and those that I experience through them, it is true. I am content.

Acknowledgments and Thanks

I wish to express my gratitude to the many people who helped me accomplish my goal of writing this book. I am fortunate. To begin with, my thanks to my Buddhist teacher, His Holiness the Seventeenth Karmapa, Ogyen Trinley Dorje. He teaches me to strive to live with genuineness and authenticity. I could not have written with vulnerability without him as my model.

I am deeply grateful to my academic teacher, Professor Charlie Hallisey, who has become one of my dearest friends over the twenty-eight years of our teacher-student relationship. Charlie transmitted to me the commitment, from his own teachers, that all learning is relational. He gifted me the rarely given lessons of how to be a humble, grateful guest and student of Buddhist teachers and texts. My thanks to Venerable Damcho, Diana Finnegan, for becoming a part of my family and teaching me the ways I can live the Dharma. Damcho discussed the entirety of my book with me and bolstered my courage along the way. Thank you to Natalie Gummer for your long friendship and intellectual partnership. I thought through many of the underlying themes in this book in conversations with her. My thanks to many women in the field of Buddhist studies who generously pointed me to resources and for their exemplary scholarship, especially to Janet Gyatso, Wendy Garling, Jan Surrey, and Natasha Heller.

Thank you to my father, David, and to my sister, Alison, who generously gave me their permission to share some of our family's most difficult moments in this book. Their similar blessing—"It's your story, you tell it how you need to"—supported me in finding my courage to tell my story. I wish to underscore and highlight the love and gratitude I feel for both of them.

To my friends near and far for love, support, and encouragement. Thank you to Sarah Schrott and Julie Rosenbaum for helping me remember my former selves with the far-sighted vision of lifelong friendships and for your professional perspectives as a psychoanalyst and physician/biomedical ethicist, respectively, which give me additional ways to interpret and understand my questions.

To my many near friends who care for my family's changing daily challenges as we live through my illness, treatment, and often severe side effects. We couldn't have gotten through many days, let alone could I have made the time to write this book, without Kelly, Simon, Steve, Kim, Sue, Julie, Tim, Fran, Vanessa, Mark, Leslie, and Gary. Leslie, thank you for sharing your professional expertise to guide me into the genre of memoir writing. Kelly, thank you for productively challenging me on my perspectives on issues of faith and for your willingness to sometimes enter into a realm of possibilities beyond the material with me. And thank you, Kelly, for your presence in my children's lives as a "second mother" now and for their future.

My thanks to the remarkable people at Wisdom Publications: to Daniel Aitken for his enthusiasm and support from the first few moments of describing this book to him and for his thoughtful insight that my illness might make rigid steps forward to publication stressful and thereby unhealthy. My thanks to Laura Cunningham, my editor, for her expert and tender care of my book; it is much better because of her suggestions.

My most love-infused thanks to my family, Ed, Ben, and Rebekah. Our family helped me find a path of love. Walking this path has been the greatest joy and source of meaning in my life; I'll walk alongside you forever.

I dedicate any merit I may generate from writing this book to people living with terminal illness and other traumas, and to their caregivers.

Bibliography: Recommended Companions

Aśvaghoṣa, and Patrick Olivelle. *Life of the Buddha*. 1st ed, New York University Press : JJC Foundation, 2008.

Dharmasena, Thera, and Obeyesekere Ranjini, trans. *Jewels of the Doctrine*. SUNY, 1991.

Diski, Jenny. *In Gratitude*. Bloomsbury, 2016.

Dobbins, James C. *Letters of the Nun Eshinni: Images of Pure Land Buddhism in Medieval Japan*. University of Hawaii Press, 2004.

Garling, Wendy. *Stars at Dawn: Forgotten Stories of Women in the Buddha's Life*. 1st edition, Shambhala, 2016.

———. "Three Forgotten Stories About the Buddha's Mother." *The Buddhist Review: TriCycle*, May 2017, https://tricycle .org/trikedaily/three-forgotten-stories-buddhas-mother.

Gtsang-smyon He-ru-ka, and Andrew Quintman. *The Life of Milarepa*. Penguin Books, 2010.

Hallisey, Charles. *Therigatha: Selected Poems of the First Buddhist Women*. Harvard University Press, 2015.

Lopez, Donald S., ed. *Buddhism in Practice*. Princeton University Press, 1995.

Nyanaponika, et al. *Great Disciples of the Buddha: Their Lives, Their Works, Their Legacy.* Wisdom Publications, 1997.

O-rgyan-'phrin-las-rdo-rje, et al. *Interconnected: Embracing Life in Our Global Society.* Wisdom Publications, 2017.

O-rgyan-'phrin-las-rdo-rje, et al. *The Heart Is Noble: Changing the World from the inside Out.* 1st edition, Shambhala, 2013.

Remnick, David. "Leonard Cohen Makes It Darker." *The New Yorker*, Oct. 2016, https://www.newyorker.com/magazine/2016/10/17/leonard-cohen-makes-it-darker.

Ricœur, Paul. *Living up to Death.* University of Chicago Press, 2009.

Rose, Gillian. *Love's Work.* New York Review Books, 2010.

Thanissaro Bhikkhu, trans. "Kucchivikara-vatthu: The Monk with Dysentery" (Mv 8.26.1–8). *Access to Insight (BCBS Edition).* Last modified November 30, 2013. https://www.accesstoinsight.org/tipitaka/vin/mv/mv.08.26.01-08.than.html.

Snyder, Gary. *Mountains and Rivers without End.* Counterpoint: Distributed by Publishers Group West, 2008.

Sontag, Susan. *Illness as Metaphor.* Farrar, Straus and Giroux, 1978.

Stewart, Jampa Mackenzie. *The Life of Gampopa: The Incomparable Dharma Lord of Tibet.* 1st ed, Snow Lion Publications, 1995.

Strong, John. "Gandhakuti: The Perfumed Chamber of the Buddha." *History of Religions*, 1977, pp. 390–406.

Umitani, Toshiyuki. "Guided by Amida Buddha." *The Taste of Nembutsu.* Honpa Hongwanji Mission of Hawaii. https://hongwanjihawaii.com/message/guided-by-amida-buddha/ Accessed October 13, 2020.

Walker, Trent. *Stirring and Stilling: A Liturgy of Cambodian*

Dharma Songs. Self-published, 2011. http://stirringandstill
ing.org.

Walters, Jonathan. "Gotami's Story." *Buddhism in Practice.* Princeton University Press, 1995, pp. 113–38.

Index

A

abuse, cycles of, 25–26
academic career, 30, 70–71, 75, 81
aging process, 16–17
AIDS, 5
Amitabha (Amida) Buddha, 7, 74,
  79–81. *See also* Sukhavati
Ananda, 104–5, 151–52, 153–55,
  156–58
anger, 26–27
  at body, 6
  at father, 99
  and fear, 34
  letting go of, 25, 102
  at mother, 33
aspirations, 52
  author's, 61, 83
  for enlightenment, 69
attachment, 126, 175
author's treatments, 64, 149,
  167–68
  brain radiation, 107–8
  brain surgery, 57–58, 63, 92–95, 117
  chemo therapy, 17, 64–65

craniotomy, 27, 89, 136, 169
  effects on body, 6
  MRI scans, 41, 42–44, 45, 65, 90,
    96, 129
  radiation, 8, 64, 72–74
  surgeries, 165–66
autonomy, expectation of, 87–88
awakened beings, 132, 145, 150, 153,
  156–57, 178
  arhats, 133
  dakinis, 44, 167
  Jizo bodhisattva, 81–82
  pratyekabuddhas, 150, 158–63
  See also Amitabha (Amida) Bud-
    dha; Buddha Shakyamuni
awareness, 55, 82, 116, 151, 173

B

beauty, being cared for by, 117
blame, 37, 66, 100
bodhichitta, 31
bodhisattvas, 68–69, 150, 158, 159,
  162–63
  Buddha as, 11, 13, 14, 15

and buddhas, relationship of,
    70–71, 133
  of compassion, 81–82
  vow of, 69–70
body
  author's relationship with, 6, 167
  at birth, 124
  Buddha's, 151
  impermanence of, 11
Buddha Shakyamuni, 11–16, 114
  intervention of, 26–27
  as model of care, 105–6
  parinirvana of, 150–55
  Prajapati and, 131–32
  prediction of becoming, 69–70,
    83
  sasana of, 158
Buddhacharita, 12–16
buddhas, 150
  as greatest field of merit, 106
  predictions of, 68–70, 71
  voice of, 83
  wisdom of, 67
  See also Amitabha Buddha; Bud-
    dha Shakyamuni, Maitreya,
    pratyekabuddhas
Buddhavamsa. See Buddhist stories: Sumedha's vow
Buddhism, 4, 55, 117. *See also* Theravada Buddhism
Buddhist practices, 74, 107–8, 116
  of Amitabha (Amida) Buddha,
    144, 145
  brahmaviharas, 160
  and faith, 140
  "Homage to the Buddha
    Amitabha" (*nembutsu*), 80

pilgrimages, 153
prayers, 73, 108, 118–19, 140
visualization practices, 74
Buddhist stories
  of Amitabha Buddha, 80
  of Ananda, 151–55
  of Buddha, 11–16, 26–27
  of Buddha's death, 132–34, 152–55
  of Buddha's mother, 57, 123,
    130–33
  on death, 173–74
  "The Demoness Kali," 25–27
  of elephant Parileyaka, 114–15
  of Eshinni and Kakushinni,
    143–45
  of Gampopa, 126–28
  Gotami Apadana, 133–34
  on grief, 122–23
  of king of Benares, 159–63
  The Life of Milarepa, 21–23, 55–56,
    127–28
  Mahaparinibbanasutta, 150–55
  Mahavastu, 104–5
  of monk Angulimala, 31–33
  prediction stories, 70, 71–72
  Sumedha's vow, 68–70, 83–84
  Therigatha, 34–36
  of Uttarakuru, 97, 98
  See also Buddhacharita;
    Dhammapada; Dharma songs
Buddhist teachings, 157–58
  on fear, 160–61
  on impermanence, 150, 151–52
  on loneliness, 164
  on motherhood, 97–99
  on preparing for death, 125

C

cancer, 6, 29, 63, 72, 88, 107
  brain, glioblastoma, 18, 66–67, 110
  living with, 82
  and loneliness, 163–65
  not fighting, 119
  as opportunity, 89
  shame for having, 110
  signs of progression, 66
  as symbol, 110
care, receiving, 87–89, 96, 104, 115–16
caregiving, 94, 105
Catholicism, 141–42
causes and conditions, 33
childhood
  abuse/trauma, 99–100
  allowing to grow, 125
  author's, 28, 116
Cohen, Leonard, 5
companionship, 111–12, 157, 158–59, 163
  of animals, 113–14, 178
  of Buddha, 150–51
  in dreams, 168, 170–71
  expectations of, 164
  to oneself, 165
  presence of, 99
  receiving care in, 109–11
  as relationships of care, 115
  in stories, 4–5, 9, 123, 166
  unique, 129
compassion, 26, 91, 105
contentment, 168, 176–77, 179
courage, 6–7, 104

D

Damcho, 49–52, 57, 59, 74, 137, 140, 173
death, 35, 66–67, 117
  acceptance of, 152
  and appreciating life, 67
  author's discovery of, 19–20
  of author's grandmother, 145–47
  of author's mother, 28–29, 155–56
  of Ed's mother, 139–40
  giving permission for, 140, 143
  and growth, 175
  little, 175
  preparing loved ones for, 125
  and remarriage, 128–29
  Siddhartha's discovery of, 13
  talking about, 116
  uncertainty of, 82–83
  as universal reality, 5
  See also under Buddhist stories
dependency, 87–88
dependent origination (*pratitya-samutpada*), 7, 52, 89, 112–13
desire, letting go of, 177
Dhammapada, 162
Dharma songs, "Khmer Lament," 130–32
diagnoses, 16, 63, 68, 116, 122, 170
dreams, 168, 170–71
Dusum Khyenpa, First Karmapa, 127

E

emotions, 36, 138. *See also* suffering
existential crisis, 18

F

faith, 61–62, 171
family relationships
attachment to, 134
author's, 74–77
with author's mother, 20–21,
24–25, 27, 30, 33–34, 88, 155–56
communion in, 142
fights, 100
response to sickness, 99
support of, 101–3
family trips, 78–80, 81–82, 117–19,
175, 176–78
fear, 5, 45–46, 48, 167–68, 169
and author's mother, 30, 34, 38,
43, 100
and anger, 27, 36, 67, 102
of becoming burden, 103, 112–13
of death, 76, 137, 159
and jealousy, 26
of king of Benares, 160–61
overcoming, 121
forgiveness, 26, 84, 132

G

Gampopa, 126–28
Gandhamadana, Mount 159–63
generosity, 165, 166
gratitude, 166, 168, 173
grief, 36, 121–26, 138
Ananda's, 156–57
for living loved ones, 126, 130,
147–48
and object of, relationship
between, 122
as storm, 121

by veneration, 153–54
without shared traditions, 142

H

Hallisey, Charlie, 29, 30, 81
Harvard Divinity School, 30
heart-mind (*citta*), 9
hospitals, 24, 27, 29, 36–37, 42–44,
77, 90, 92–96, 107–9, 129
See also author's treatments

I

identity, holding, 35
Illness as Metaphor (Sontag), 110
illusions, 6, 59, 76, 135, 155
imagination, 3–4, 7, 23, 48, 56, 57,
140, 167
impermanence, 4, 11, 39, 75–76, 84,
121, 131, 136, 167
acknowledging one's own, 138
and illness, 122
of life, 19, 28
and love, 137
offerings of, 101, 126
In Gratitude (Diski), 5–6
independence, giving up, 88
India, 51, 55, 56
*Interconnected: Embracing Life in
Our Global Society* (Seventeenth Karmapa), 61

J

Jewish practices, 138, 146
Jizo, 81–82
Jodo Shinshu Buddhism, 4

K

karma, 67, 106, 160
Kisa Gotami, 102

L

Land of Bliss. *See* Sukhavati
life
  as companionship, 115
  and death, dialogue between, 143
  letting go of, 139
  stages of, 129–30
  time frame of, 72
Living Up to Death (Ricoeur), 122
loneliness, 17, 154, 155, 163, 164–65
love, 147
  orienting toward, 9, 107
  unconditional, 135–36, 137
Love's Work (Rose), 5

M

Maitreya, 158
Marpa, 56
Masatoshi Nagatomi, 7
Maya. *See* Buddhist stories: of
  Buddha's mother
memories, 67
Meru, Mount, 97
mindfulness practice, 73
Mingyur Rinpoche, 125
monastics, 54, 104–6, 114–15,
  152–53, 156–57, 160–61. *See also*
  nuns; *Therigatha*
mother(s), 98
  abuse by, 99–100
  all people as, 97

author as, 36–39, 75–77, 85–86,
  112, 123–25, 135–36, 174–75
Milarepa's, 22–23
See also under Buddhist stories;
  family relationships

N

New York Times, 167
The New Yorker, 5
nirvana, 12, 132, 150
nuns, 8, 132–33

O

Ogyen Trinley Dorje, Seventeenth
  Karmapa, 31, 50–57, 58–62, 80,
  85, 89–90, 101, 169, 170
oncologists, 63, 68

P

paradox, 157
parinirvana, 133, 150, 162
personal development, 87
poetry, 84–85, 175–76
post-surgery, 95–96, 122
Prajapati, 57, 131–32, 150
pratyekabuddhas, 150, 158–63
pregnancy, author's, 46–47
privilege, 106–7

R

reading
  with empathy, 22–23
  as practice, 8–9, 23, 59, 138, 144,
    163
Reality, 168
rebirth, 54, 67, 140, 144, 145

relics, 153
renunciation, 15
rituals
  as container for compassion, 141
  family, 174
  for grieving, 142
  between living and dead, 140–41

S

self, sense of, 95
self-sufficiency, losing, 95–96
"Sevenfold Cause and Effect," 31
shame, 31, 110
Shobogenzo (Dogen), 117
Siddhartha Gautama. *See* Buddha
  Shakyamuni
spiritual friend (*kalyanamitra*),
  49, 137
  See also Damcho
spiritual teacher, author's con-
  nection to. *See* Ogyen Trinley
  Dorje, Seventeenth Karmapa
Strong, John, 154
suffering, 11, 16, 29, 102, 119, 165
Sukhavati, 81, 144, 145, 169

T

teacher, author's time as, 84, 87
terminal illness, 65, 88–89

Theravada Buddhism, 4, 70–71, 97,
  130, 152–55, 159
Therigatha, 7–8, 34, 49
Tibetan Buddhism, 4
time, author's experience of, 84–85
trauma, 30, 99–100, 117
Tsongkhapa, 30, 31
tumor, 18, 27, 43, 46, 63, 110

U

uncertainty, accepting, 68

V

vulnerability, 6, 75, 96, 104, 105

W

"With This Flesh" (Snyder), 84–85

Y

Yashodhara, 132–33, 150
Yellow Finches (Derris), 176

Z

Zen Buddhism, 117

About the Author

D r. Karen Derris is a scholar of South and Southeast Asian Buddhist traditions and professor of religious studies at the University of Redlands. Her research focuses on the intersection of literature and feminist ethics in pre-modern Buddhist traditions, particularly focusing upon the central importance of community in Buddhist ethical and spiritual development. Dr. Derris received her PhD from the Committee on the Study of Religion at Harvard University in 2000.

What to Read Next
from Wisdom Publications

Interconnected
Embracing Life in Our Global Society
The Karmapa, Ogyen Trinley Dorje

"We are now so interdependent that it is in our own interest to take the whole of humanity into account. Hope lies with the generation who belong to the twenty-first century. If they can learn from the past and shape a different future, later this century the world could be a happier, more peaceful, and more environmentally stable place. I am very happy to see in this book the Karmapa Rinpoche taking a lead and advising practical ways to reach this goal." —His Holiness the Dalai Lama

Zen Cancer Wisdom
Tips for Making Each Day Better
Daju Suzanne Friedman

"This book has become one of my most valuable resources. It's a rich and comprehensive guide to opening our minds to our life as it is and for soothing our struggling bodies."
—Toni Bernhard, author of *How to Be Sick*

How to Be Sick
A Buddhist-Inspired Guide for the Chronically Ill and Their Caregivers
Toni Bernhard
Foreword by Sylvia Boorstein

Updated with new insights and practices hard-won from Toni's own ongoing life experience, this is a must-read for anyone who is—or who might one day be—sick.

Bearing the Unbearable
Love, Loss, and the Heartbreaking Path of Grief
Joanne Cacciatore

"Simultaneously heartwrenching and uplifting. Cacciatore offers practical guidance on coping with profound and life-changing grief. This book is destined to be a classic . . . [it] is simply the best book I have ever read on the process of grief."
—Ira Israel, *The Huffington Post*

Awake at the Bedside
Contemplative Teachings on Palliative and End-of-Life Care
Edited by Koshin Paley Ellison and Matty Weingast

"The greatest degree of inner tranquility comes from the development of love and compassion. The more we care for the happiness of others, the greater is our own sense of well-being. Cultivating a close, warmhearted feeling for others automatically puts the mind at ease. It is the ultimate source of success in life. *Awake at the Bedside* supports this development of love and compassion."
—His Holiness the Dalai Lama

About Wisdom Publications

Wisdom Publications is the leading publisher of classic and contemporary Buddhist books and practical works on mindfulness. To learn more about us or to explore our other books, please visit our website at wisdomexperience.org or contact us at the address below.

Wisdom Publications
199 Elm Street
Somerville, MA 02144 USA

We are a 501(c)(3) organization, and donations in support of our mission are tax deductible.

Wisdom Publications is affiliated with the Foundation for the Preservation of the Mahayana Tradition (FPMT).